D1486347

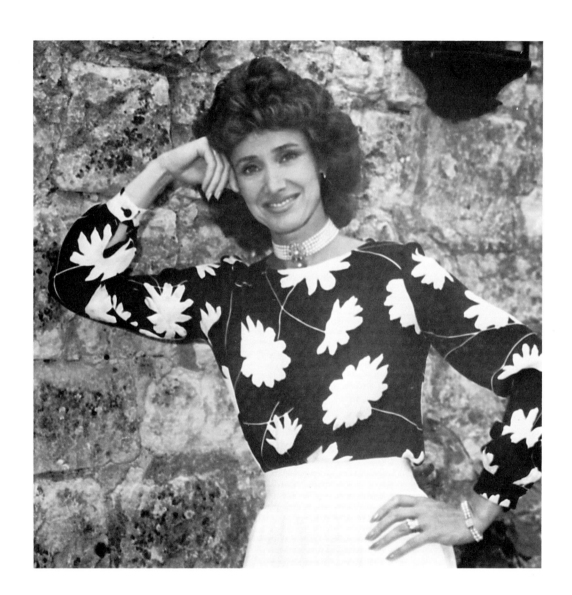

Jan Leeming

simply looking good

GUILD PUBLISHING
LONDON

This edition published 1984 by
Book Club Associates
by arrangement with Weidenfeld & Nicolson

Copyright © 1984 by Jan Leeming

Illustrations by Ann Vincent

Printed in Great Britain by
Butler & Tanner Ltd, Frome and London

Contents

To my loved ones
for all their patience and understanding

Author's Acknowledgments

I would like to thank the following for their assistance in creating *Simply Looking Good*. My editor, Hilary Arnold, for her encouragement, enthusiasm and hard work, and for keeping me on the right track. Edward St Maur who is a kind and superb photographer. He took the trouble to understand me and has portrayed me as I see myself. Thanks to his assistant Gilly as well. Andrew Kay, the designer, who made very hard work great fun, gained my trust and bullied me throughout. My hairdresser of many years, Jean Mays, who is also a dear friend, for her constant devotion and moral support and for her help with the chapter on hair. Claire Hunt for her advice and information on physiology. Clare Maxwell Hudson for allowing me to use some of her cosmetic recipes. Celia Hunter for her help with the chapter on make-up. Sally Ann Voak for her advice on diet and exercise. Pauline Hedges who typed my manuscript and encouraged me. Many thanks to Pat, Patricia, Eva and June who allowed me to restyle their appearance, and to Mrs Ed Kyle-Price for the use of her home.

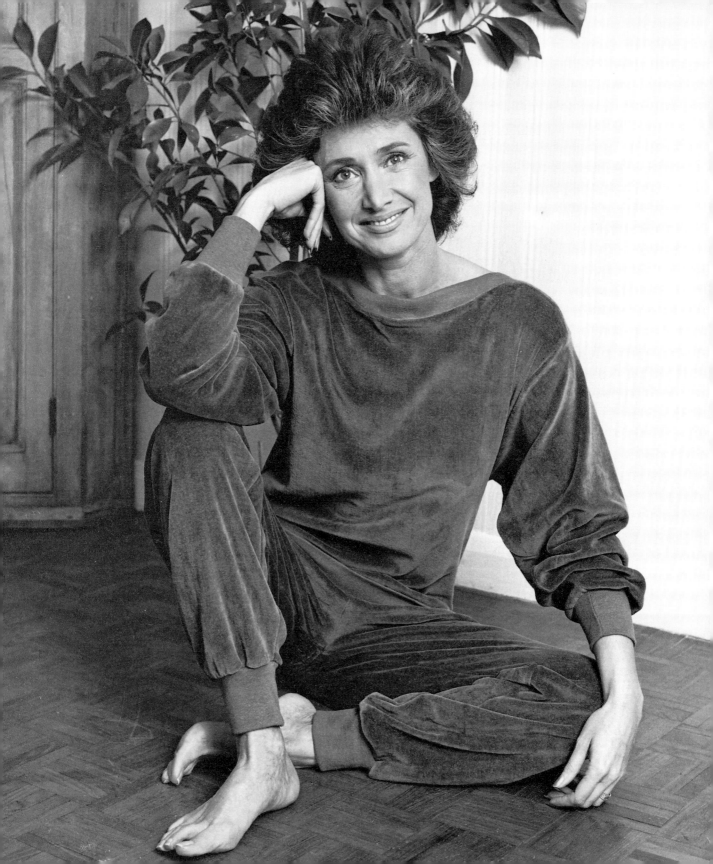

Introduction

There are millions of women like me — taking care of a family and home whilst working in a demanding but enjoyable job. My career in television has spanned twenty-two years and for eighteen of those I was happily working in regional television. I was sometimes recognized by viewers but generally regarded as 'the girl next door'. All that changed when I started reading the national news on BBC television. I had heard people in television talking about 'living in a goldfish bowl' and I soon discovered what they meant. Now it is as if I am always on parade, always on duty, and people always notice how I look and what I am wearing.

This is somewhat daunting to me since I do not have hours to spend pampering myself. Managing a growing toddler, running a house and holding down a career leaves me with only snatched moments in which to take stock of my appearance.

I care about the way I look, not only because of my job; it is a fundamental aspect of my personality. Vanity no doubt plays a part in this but I believe it is something I share with most women — you feel more relaxed and confident if you know you look as good as possible.

When I was asked to write a style and beauty book I was extremely flattered but my immediate reaction was that I did not have the necessary qualifications for the task. After all, such books are written either by professional beauticians or by exceptionally lovely and glamorous stars. They usually propose complicated beauty routines and make-up suggestions, or contain a succession of exhausting exercises. Generally they seem to imply that we should devote an enormous amount of time and energy to our looks. As a working mother, I do not have the time to indulge in such practices. Oh that I did! A lengthy session in the bathroom each day, followed by an hour's workout and a quick shower, before applying a fabulous face, is out of the question for me — and for most of you no doubt. My professional knowledge is limited to what I have picked up over the years, and I am certainly not a great beauty. How come I wrote the book? Simply because I felt there was nothing available for women like me.

What I can share with you is my knowledge of how to make the very best of yourself without devoting a large portion of your life to your appearance. I have to look my best, and I know I do not always achieve it, but over the years I have developed a simple approach to the problem, nothing too demanding, and a system which has become second nature to me. My skin-care routine is fast and as automatic as brushing my teeth. I apply my make-up equally quickly and the amount I wear depends on circumstances. I have virtually no time at all for clothes shopping so I have had to discipline myself to maintain a flexible, co-ordinated wardrobe. A healthy diet is essential to one's looks so, mainly through trial and error, I have worked out what I should eat to ensure my intake is balanced and nutritional.

I do not have time for exercise but I am well aware of the advantages of doing so. Were it not for the fact that I exert a vast amount of physical energy in my daily routine I would certainly take regular exercise.

'That's all very well,' I can hear you saying, 'but she works in television and no doubt has an army of beauticians, make-up artists and wardrobe assistants at her beck and call.' Not true. I apply my own make-up for the screen and do my own hair, visiting a trusted provincial hairdresser on average once every six weeks. I wear my own clothes on television. Obviously I cannot dress sloppily or outrageously, and there are basic rules about colour that have to be adhered to because cameras react badly to some shades.

I am in no position to write a gospel on beauty and style, to be followed to the letter. This book is intended as a practical handbook to make you more complete and attractive. I particularly hope it will benefit women who feel they are beyond a time in their lives when they can face aerobics, strict diets, exotic make-up and the dictates of high fashion.

Not so long ago women were written off at thirty-five and regarded as beyond the pale by forty-five. My generation have much to be grateful for. Today a woman over thirty-five knows she has come of age rather than regretting she is beginning to age. She has a new-found freedom, she is her own woman, knows what she likes and dislikes. She may have chosen to raise a family or follow a career, and very likely she has done both. She could have married in her teens or her late thirties, may have started a family at twenty-four or forty-two. She is probably past worrying too much about what others think of her and controls her own destiny.

Given all this, it is obviously never too late to start taking a really positive attitude to your looks. One thing never changes and that is that as we get older our bodies show signs of ageing. Skin care, make-up, clothes and diet are more important as the years go by. If you have neglected yourself for a long time – allowed the sun to wreak havoc with your skin, have been too busy to bother with stylish clothes – it is probably because your energy has been put into caring for others, be it a family or a boss, or because you have not stopped to think of the consequences of neglecting your looks. You cannot put the clock back but you can certainly slow it down.

I cannot, unfortunately, provide a secret formula to make you look like Sophia Loren or Raquel Welch, Brit Ekland or Joan Collins. I think I can help you maximize your good points and minimize the bad. Most important of all, I hope I can encourage and inform. A decent outer shell is a bonus and naturally gorgeous people have a distinct advantage. But a decent outer shell is not hard to achieve no matter what nature provides.

However, you can be as attractive as possible yet not achieve beauty in the true sense. It is a cliché but beauty does come to some extent from within. An outgoing, optimistic, sparkling personality has a head start in looking good. And most of the world's great beauties would concur that you can be more attractive over thirty-five than earlier in life.

It is a Golden Age – make the most of it.

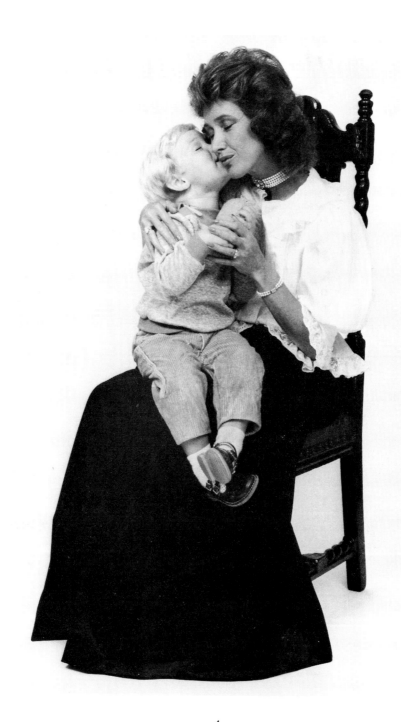

4

Self-Assessment

Given ideal circumstances, pots of money and oodles of time, it would be possible to indulge in all the things which are beyond my reach, and the reach of the vast majority of women. Anyone would get thoroughly bored with too much self-indulgence, but for a while it would be the height of luxury to be able to go to the professionals and find out how best to improve one's looks.

I would visit a top beauty salon and take expensive treatments to improve my skin, my body and my hair. I would then head for a fashion consultant, if such people exist, to get the up-to-the-minute information on fashion shapes and colours and to discuss how I can combine them with my own style. I'd then spend several days wandering from one exclusive store to the next, selecting a wardrobe of beautiful, flattering clothes for the next season.

By the time I had chosen exquisite accessories to match my designer clothes, I would no doubt be exhausted, so off I'd go to a good health spa. There I would take full advantage of their expertise and equipment in order to clean out my system and thoroughly relax.

Back home, and no doubt feeling and looking wonderful, I would keep up the good work by undertaking a series of keep-fit or dance classes, to be taken at my leisure so that I slowly build up my strength and tone my body. I would also visit a good nutritionist in order that an expert could analyse my present diet and suggest the best way for me to eat to ensure maximum nutrition and health.

I would investigate relaxation techniques and find out how to remove stress from my life as much as possible. Finally, I would take a long and luxurious holiday, to complete my personal overhaul.

Sweet dreams!

In reality, if you do decide you need a personal overhaul, your life does not conveniently stop so that you can undertake a programme of pampering and self-indulgence. The overhaul has to be squeezed in to your normal schedule of daily living. For most of us this is extremely hectic – looking after children, working, running a home. And even if the time could be found, the budget does not stretch to health spas, expensive beauty parlours or professional nutritionists, not to mention designer clothes.

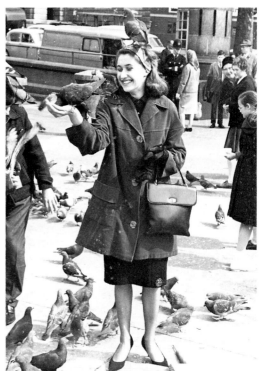

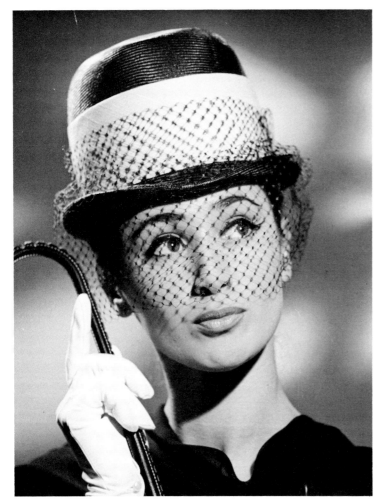

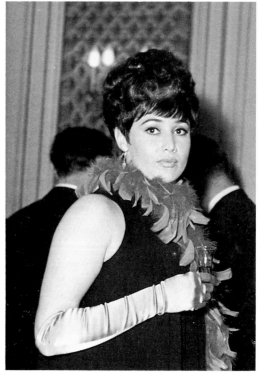

The biggest bonus, I believe, which one would get from a really expensive and thorough overhaul would be professional advice. Experts in the art of looking good and being healthy would consider you and your lifestyle and suggest ways of improving both! Half the battle is won when you know what action is necessary and where improvements can be made.

Given that most of us can only dream of obtaining the full range of top professional help, then we have to undertake their role ourselves. This must begin with a thorough self-assessment. Do what the experts would do – stand back and take a long hard look at yourself.

Put aside a few hours and make sure you will not be interrupted. Place yourself in front of a full-length mirror with pen and paper to hand. Choose a time when life is not too hectic otherwise you will not be able to concentrate fully. Do it before a holiday rather than immediately after one, when you are probably relaxed, suntanned and looking better anyway. Ensure that you are dressed as you would be normally during the day, having applied your usual make-up.

You are going to be brutally frank with yourself and as objective as possible. It is extremely difficult to be objective about yourself so you will have to work at it. You probably have general feelings about your appearance which you have kept for a long time – put them out of your mind. No doubt you have an ideal of how you would like to look and you admire particular women in public life who, you think, live up to that ideal. Put your ideal image out of your mind also. Stand well back and take a fresh look at someone you do not often stand back from – yourself.

Now take that long hard look, and keep looking. Try and sum up what you see and note it down. Make a general assessment such as 'tired and shabby', 'healthy but no style', 'pretty but old-fashioned'. Imagine you are your own best friend and be constructive.

Slowly consider all of you, from head to toe, and as you go through write down all that you consider to be negative features or areas with room for improvement. Include permanent defects – we all have them. My biggest defects are obvious ageing, a lined neck and veined feet. The ageing speaks for itself. My neck has been lined since I was in my mid-teens and when I was younger some people were kind enough to refer to the lines as my 'beauty bracelets' – rubbish! There is nothing beautiful about them. They are the result of a teenage thyroid problem and my fine skin which goes crêpey at the neck. My feet bother me even more. Because of bad circulation, I have a hideous network of small broken veins which I can neither disguise nor get rid of completely. I have to accept that I cannot go without tights in summer and no one is going to kiss my feet.

You may consider aspects of yourself as defects when they are not, so look carefully. For instance, if you have always longed to be curvaceous but have small breasts, look at your whole self and consider whether they are out of proportion. If not they are hardly a defect. Think of the number of women who would note in this category that they have sagging breasts which spoil the line of their clothes. Small breasts can be a bonus. Similarly, you may be obsessed with the size of your thighs – many women are. Again, consider if they are out of proportion. Do they really bulge from your hips or are you generally overweight. Look again; is it not that you merely have a full figure?

Consider your shape. Study the diagrams showing the various builds of women. You may not obviously fit totally into any one of these but see which one is your approximate shape. Most of us are a combination of shapes.

Look at your hairstyle and make-up. Do they flatter you and make the best of your face? Does your hair need restyling and is it shining and healthy or lank and tired? Should your eyes be emphasized and is that lipstick an attractive shade for your colouring?

What about your clothes? Do they suit you, make the best of your figure and are they co-ordinated or merely thrown together? Do not forget your feet. Do your shoes complement what you are wearing and flatter your legs?

As you go through the bad points, keep your distance from the mirror and only write down what you see, not what you have always thought. I have a friend who is convinced she has fat ankles and is self-conscious about her legs. In fact, I would never consider her to have fat ankles and if she would do the mirror test she would see, hopefully, that they do not stand out as a defect.

Note whether your posture is good and if you look healthy. Does stress and strain show in your face and body? Smile and look at your teeth, and also note the quality of your hands.

The next stage of self-assessment is equally difficult and requires just as much objectivity. Consider all the things you like about yourself and regard as good points. You may have noted your hairstyle as a negative but the hair itself may be one of your best features – thick and luxuriant, but badly cut. You may have good bone structure; an attractive, well proportioned figure; good legs or lovely hands.

When you have finished your notes, study them slowly. Start to consider how you might improve the defects and capitalize on good points. Why is your skin sallow? Is it because you eat the wrong things, because you are overtired or because you take no care of it? If you have noted your stomach protrudes, has it anything to do with wearing a tight belt or holding yourself badly? The bags under your eyes could be the result of too many late nights, sinus problems or simply getting older.

Are you making the best of your assets? Is a pretty face with good skin spoiled by too severe a hairstyle or bad teeth? If your clothes skimmed your hips rather than clung to them would that take away unpleasant bulges?

You may be pleased with your figure because you have successfully lost weight or have always been slim and maintain it by eating as little as possible. But has this

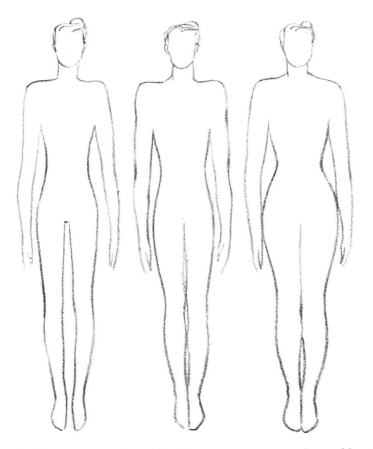

Body shapes
LEFT TO RIGHT
Ectomorph, slim and angular with little excess fat; mesomorph, large bones, broad shoulders and more muscle than fat; endomorph, narrower but with wide hips, and a tendency to plumpness.

lead to a generally unhealthy appearance and would a few extra pounds on the body not fill out that face and make it look younger? We are obsessed by being slim but being too thin can lead to as many problems as excess weight. However, if you do feel you are overweight, consider why. Is it a sedentary occupation and too many cream cakes? Has your metabolism been slowed down by endless diets followed by endless binges? Or do you simply have the figure of Marilyn Monroe but have always longed to be a Twiggy? If this is so, then face up to the fact that no amount of dieting and aerobics will achieve your desires and make the most of what you have – a gorgeous body. Think about dressing to show off your curves rather than dieting to get rid of them – you won't. You cannot change the basic shape of your body frame.

Take a little time to consider what you eat. There has been so much publicity about eating correctly that one inevitably gets terribly confused. At one moment we pop as many vitamin pills as we can swallow only to find soon afterwards that

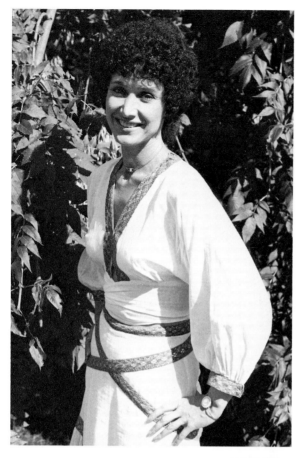

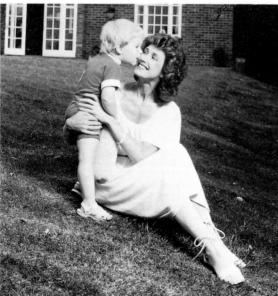

LEFT
An Afro hairstyle and classical Grecian costume . . .

. . . immediately followed by a homely, no-nonsense look in 1980.

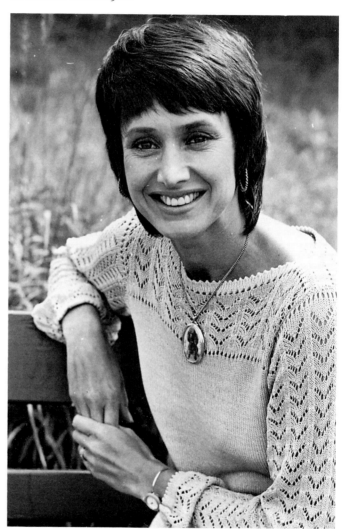

LEFT
1983 and quite a different look again with Jonathan in the garden.

someone is claiming they do no good. Eat lots of high fibre food, we are told, and the rest will take care of itself. Then suddenly the great enemy is salt which you have been shaking liberally on to raw vegetables in order to enjoy them. Generally, though, you know if your diet is basically healthy or unhealthy. The chapter on food will help you decide, but after the mirror test is a good time to make a general assessment, particularly if you have any doubts about your eating habits and how they are affecting your appearance.

Other aspects which can seriously affect your appearance are stress and tiredness. If you feel run down and unhappy you may not realize that it can make your hair lifeless, your skin sallow and removes the inner glow that is an aid to looking good. Feeling negative about yourself is a sure way of not looking your best. If your general assessment was poor when you looked in that mirror, and if you have before you a long list of bad points and few good ones, then you feel badly about yourself. It may be for good reason and your notes may initiate some positive changes. However, if your mirror test is reflecting a general depression, or the stress in your life, or the fact that you are basically exhausted, or even that you are downright bored with your life and yourself, then you may be tempted now to see the mirror test as another affirmation of the fact that things are bad. We all know the old adage that if one is feeling low then rushing out to buy a new lipstick or popping into the hairdresser for a restyle will make things better. It's old but nonetheless true. And it can be taken to a logical conclusion. If merely buying a new lipstick makes you feel a little better, then consider what a complete overhaul of your appearance will do. If you are depressed and tired, and unhappy with your appearance, then finish your mirror test with a promise to yourself that you will take steps to start remedying the matter. Do that and you will probably, hopefully, feel better already. You are now on the correct path to looking better.

If you have carried out the mirror test correctly, you should have realized which aspects of your appearance require action. If you have been honest with yourself, you will probably have discovered that there is room for improvement in most areas – complexion, make-up, diet, exercise and clothes. Some may require more action than others, but you should be prepared to rethink your attitude to just about everything that goes towards making an attractive you. The hardest part is over, so now let's get down to simply looking good.

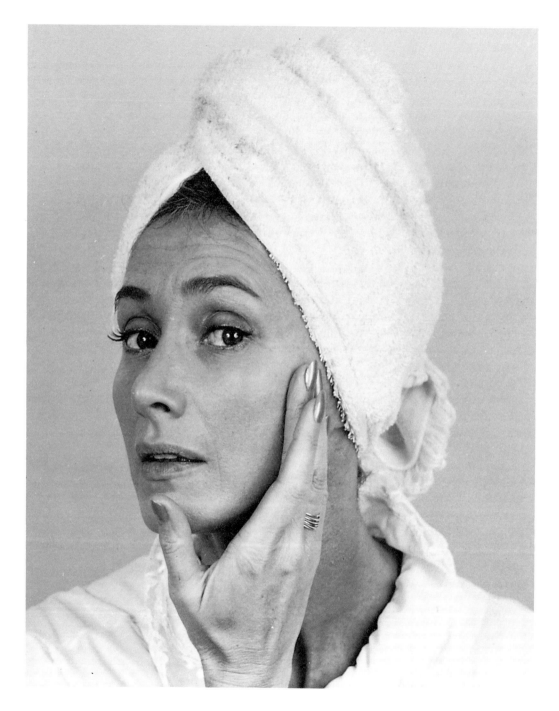

Skin Care

Y ou are what you eat and your complexion reflects your diet. Reorganizing your eating habits takes time and I am sure you are impatient to deal with the part of you which is most visible and vulnerable – your face. However, do not think you can skip the chapter on food – do so at your peril!

Most of us have neglected ourselves hoping that youth would last forever and our skin take care of itself. Did you bother with moisturizers, night creams and neck massage in your early twenties? Of course you did not – neither did I. Did you overdo the time in the sun to get a glorious sexy tan? I did too. Do you drink alcohol, smoke cigarettes or adore chocolate? If none of those apply to you then you are lucky indeed and your skin has probably benefited.

It is no good looking back with heavy regrets – the damage we did to our skins, or are still doing, cannot be undone but it is never too late to start slowing down the ageing process and increasing the amount of care we give our complexions. Ideally we should all have started in our teens.

Of course there are exceptions to every rule and there are women who have superb complexions throughout their lives. You are bound to know, and I certainly do, friends who wash their face with ordinary soap and water, never show it to a beauty cream, and still have lovely skin. But they are the exceptions.

There is no simple answer as to why some complexions are better than others, but heredity plays a part. Take a particularly lovely 'English rose' such as Katie Boyle – a beautiful woman with a wonderful skin. I asked once, during an interview, what her secret was. She believed it was due to the fact that despite her English rose image she is of Italian extraction. So she may well have an oilier complexion than is usual for British women. Of course, Katie Boyle looks after her skin but she does start with a distinct advantage over those with particularly fine and dry skin. Fine skin wrinkles more easily and more rapidly than oilier skin. However, it is not as likely to break out in spots and it takes make-up more easily.

Most of the model girls used in cosmetic advertisements or on the beauty pages of magazines appear to have superb complexions too. Of course there are tricks used to assist the image – lighting, make-up, the way the camera has been focused and so on. But the most obvious reason that they appear so gorgeous is that they are very young. Do not try and compete or believe that creams and lotions will transform your face into a face which advertises skin-care products. That would require a miracle.

Why skin ages

I am not going to both confuse and bore you with endless details of the skin's construction, layers, cells and so on. For our purposes, what is important is that skin ages and when it does it shows. We have to look at why this happens and learn how best to slow down the ageing process as much as possible.

Exposure to the elements

It has been said that if the human face were never exposed to the sun, wind, air and so on, that it would remain as smooth and glowing as a baby's forever. Hard to believe and not really very comforting, especially for those of us who have not only exposed it but roasted it to a golden brown as often as possible. The sun is the number one enemy in the fight against ageing skin. It dries it out, kills off important elements in the skin's composition, can cause serious problems and is generally destructive.

It is worth looking around the world and back into history for confirmation of this. Our great-great-grandmothers took enormous care not to expose their faces to the elements. They were looking after their complexions because in those Victorian days a weathered skin indicated that a woman had a hard life in the open. As far as social status was concerned it meant you were of the lower order. Sun-tans first became fashionable, and desirable, in the 1920s when mad young things discovered the joys of the beach and of escaping to southerly climes to enjoy warm weather. Such expeditions were beyond the reach of the vast majority of people, so suddenly a sun-tan became an indication of wealth and prosperity, just as porcelain whiteness had been previously.

One only has to study the faces of people who live in a hot climate, particularly if they originate from cooler areas of the world, to see the harmful effects of the sun. The skin may have a wonderful tan but it is usually leather-like in texture, covered in dark splotches which hardly pass as mere freckles, and is highly wrinkled. I lived in Australia for a while where the sun is extremely strong. Skin cancer is a serious problem there, and so is leathery skin. Most Australian women are now well aware of the damaging effects of the sun-tan obsession but they learnt the hard way. I admit that I loved being well tanned when I was there but I truly regret it now.

It is advisable always to wear a sun-filter cream if you are going to expose your face to the sun – even if you also wear a sun-hat. A golden tan does look lovely on the face, and is a great confidence booster. As you get older, do not risk the damage of natural sun-tanning but use a tanning lotion if you want to be brown. Perhaps you have tried them and have been horrified by the false effect some of them can have and by streaking. However, today modern scientific methods are producing excellent self-tanning products which do look natural. They are quite expensive but think of the money you are saving in filter creams, since they usually contain sun-filters, and in anti-wrinkle treatments later on.

Dehydration

We are told constantly that our skin requires moisture and moisture means only one thing – water. The skin naturally contains a high water content but as one gets older it tends to dry out more easily and become dehydrated; dry skin is thirsty skin. Water is held in the skin by an oily protective layer of a substance called sebum which is excreted from glands below the skin's surface. The glands tend to be less efficient year by year, so the water in the skin evaporates more and more easily. As the skin dries out it is more likely to wrinkle and feel taut.

In order to avoid dehydration you must avoid situations where the skin is going to become dried out; ensure that you maintain a protective layer on the surface of the skin to lock in the moisture; and replace the water lost. There are many situations in which the environment is such that it dries out your skin. Obviously bright sunshine and hot, dry weather is one. In winter months, spending long hours inside with the central-heating turned up is equally damaging. Humidifiers replace the moisture in the air of a heated room and are well worth having. Alternatively, a few open bowls of water set around a room have a similar effect. A spray mister – either one used for plants and using tap water or, preferably, a spray-can containing mineral water, is also a great help in hot, dry situations. Spray the face regularly to keep it moist.

Some drugs are extremely dehydrating, including antihistamines used against hay fever and in cold 'cures'. Alcohol is dehydrating as well as being bad for your skin in other ways – one of its most serious effects, if a great deal is consumed, is that it causes broken capillaries which show as tiny red veins on the face. At worst, alcohol leads to constantly bloodshot eyes and a swollen, red nose. If you do drink in moderation, also take plenty of water to compensate for the dehydration. Coffee is also dehydrating.

Drinking plenty of water generally helps with dehydration and resulting dry skin, so try and replace some of the less desirable drinks you take during the day with a glass of cold water.

We replace the water lost from the skin with moisturizers. The water they contain passes into the skin and the creamy texture of moisturizing products enables us to smooth them onto the skin. Moisturizers also contain some oil to help create that protective layer on the surface and lock in the moisture. However, if the skin is clogged with dirt or has a dry, flaky surface, the moisturizer will not be adequately absorbed by the skin and the surface will hold the water and oil where it will soon evaporate. Clogged pores, dirt and dry patches are also preventing glands beneath the skin's surface from releasing the natural protection of sebum. Thorough cleansing is essential to ensure that the pores are clear and your skin is able to absorb a moisturizer. If you believe that you are drying your skin by cleaning it – unless you are scrubbing the surface and using harsh detergents found in most soaps – then you are wrong. On the contrary, you are wasting time and money if you apply moisturizer to skin which is not completely clean.

Elasticity

Take a piece of skin on the back of your hand between your thumb and forefinger and watch how quickly it springs back. The older you get, the longer it will take, and if you never bother with hand lotions it will take longer still. The skin's natural elasticity lessens with age and there is little we can do to avoid it but much we can do to slow down the process.

The skin contains proteins which support it and help maintain its elastic quality. Collagen is perhaps the best-known of these proteins. As we get older, the amount of collagen in the skin lessens and is not reproduced, so the skin is less elastic and the cells are not naturally plumped out. The sun kills off collagen in the skin – it really is an enemy in every possible way. Vitamin C is important for maintaining collagen so an intake of vitamin tablets can help. Smoking and drinking alcohol deplete the Vitamin C in the body, so cutting them down, or out, is strongly recommended.

Many products on the market, generally in the form of moisturizers, night creams or firming creams, contain proteins to help supplement those we have lost and keep the skin elastic and plump. If you are able to afford it, you can have collagen injected under the skin to help with serious lines around the eyes or between nose and mouth.

Rejuvenation

The top layer of your facial skin is dead. As new cells are formed below the surface they push away the dead cells on the top, and in this way your skin constantly rejuvenates. I hate to keep repeating those awful words 'as you get older' yet again, but with increasing years, the skin rejuvenates less efficiently. The skin tends to either become sallow and dull, or dry and flaky, because the dead cells linger on the surface. Your natural glow is lost beneath them.

In order to aid the natural rejuvenating process, regular exfoliating, or sloughing, of the dead cells is necessary. It not only greatly improves the appearance of the skin but helps your skin fight the other ageing processes. The layer of dead cells counteracts the protective layer on the surface which locks in moisture. Dead cells prevent the products you apply to your face from being absorbed. They block pores and hinder cleansing.

Wrinkles

Given that ageing skin dehydrates more easily, is less elastic and does not rejuvenate efficiently, it tends to wrinkle and sag. In addition, with age our eyes often become sunken, our gums shrink and our skin stretches. Wrinkles are the most obvious sign of ageing but they go hand in hand with these other developments on the face.

Make-up can help counteract some aspects of ageing but it requires a healthy complexion for it to be most effective and too heavily applied it actually accentuates wrinkles. Most wrinkles are expression lines which form when we smile, talk, frown and so on. They become permanent as you get older. You may not realize just how much you furrow your brow or wrinkle your nose during the day, and even while you sleep. However, to suggest that you adopt a mask-like expression at all times to avoid wrinkles is not only absurd but almost counter-productive. As I have said, perhaps the best antidote to a few wrinkles is a sparkling personality and all the facial expressions that go with it. But it is good to remember that expression lines caused by laughing are far more attractive on the face than those caused by frowning. Stress is bad for you, obviously – it makes you feel lousy. It also affects your skin and hair, and your wrinkles. If you are particularly tense and worried, you may frown through the night.

If you are aware of the ageing processes I have described and you take action to deal with them, then you are taking action against wrinkles. Specific anti-wrinkle creams are designed to add protein and moisture to the skin and plump out the cells but it is equally important to avoid the sun and exfoliate the skin. Wrinkle creams used alone are wasted – they should be used as part of your beauty routine, not as a last-minute, desperate attempt to halt ageing. If the wrinkles are already there, no amount of cream will actually remove them. However, if you care for your skin then less wrinkles will form.

Your skin type

It is essential to follow a regular and thorough skin-care routine. The right products will cleanse your skin and help replace the natural proteins, oils and water lost from it, as well as nourishing the existing cells. The products you use must be correct for your particular skin type or else they will not have the right effect and could cause problems. So what is your skin type? If you are not sure – do the tissue test.

Tissue test

Thoroughly cleanse your skin at night and ensure that your hair is fixed away from your face while you sleep. In the morning, in front of a natural light source, preferably next to a window, look into a mirror. Take a piece of tissue paper, not the kind used in boxes of tissues but the crisper version used to pack clothes or china, and hold it over your face. Press it gently into your skin section by section around the face. Press over the left side of your face, around the nose, under the chin and down the neck. Now repeat down the right side of your face.

When you remove the tissue look at it carefully. All greasy areas will show as oily patches on the tissue paper. If the grease shows overall you have a definitely greasy

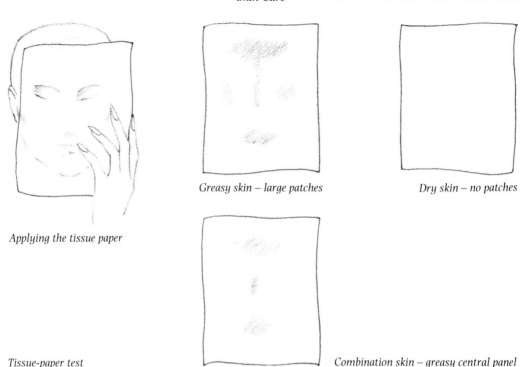

Applying the tissue paper

Greasy skin – large patches

Dry skin – no patches

Tissue-paper test

Combination skin – greasy central panel

skin. More likely, you will have greasy patches, and these will most probably be found along the centre of the face – around the chin, nose and forehead. If the cheeks and neck do not show as greasy at all, and only the central area comes out as a greasy patch, then you have a combination skin. If the entire paper remains clean then your skin is normal or dry, and most likely dry if you are over thirty-five.

Greasy skin

The skin is greasy because it produces too much sebum. Sebum is the substance which forms a natural protective layer on the skin's surface to protect the skin and keep in its moisture. Sebum is excreted by glands below the skin's surface and when there is over-production of sebum other problems can occur – open pores, black heads and sallow skin. If you have greasy skin it may be coarse, thick and shiny. You may find that your foundation tends to turn orangey in colour and you will almost definitely have greasy hair.

Dry skin

The opposite of over-production of sebum, a lack of it, causes the skin's tissues to dry out since the protective layer of sebum is not sufficient to keep in the moisture. You may find that it feels taut and tends to produce dry, flaky patches, both on the face and body. Your elbows and knees will probably be dry. Fine lines around your eyes and mouth may have appeared when you were relatively young, and frown lines on the forehead could be pronounced. Your neck is another problem area if you have dry skin, and your skin may have a pink tinge.

Combination skin

Perhaps the most common of all for people in northern areas of Europe is combination skin. The middle panel can be quite greasy, with the cheeks and neck tending to be dry. Spots will tend to break out in the central panel while lines are a problem elsewhere.

Sensitive skin

Sensitive skin can be slightly greasy and tend to become inflamed but more commonly it is a result of very thin and dry skin which reddens easily when irritated by the weather or by cosmetics.

Simple beauty routine

I will now go through the basics of a beauty routine, distinguishing skin types. What follows is a fast and simple system so take the time to study it carefully and then prepare to add the system to your daily routine.

Cleansing is the first essential and at night it is particularly important. A few minutes at the end of the day can take years off your appearance. Yet I am staggered by the number of women who own up to going to bed without cleansing their faces. Even if you wear no, or very little, make-up, night cleansing should be a priority. Look around you at the damage that grime and pollution inflict on hard stone buildings. Now give another thought to your poor fragile face. By the end of each day, whether you live in town or country, you have a layer of grime on your face. That dirt is having a field day clogging up the pores of your skin, eating away at it. In addition, you probably have a layer of make-up and even more likely you have several layers, added to during the day.

I am lazy about many things but my one golden rule is that no matter how tired I am or how late it is, I go through my night cleansing routine. It takes me five minutes each night: whether I have been at home all day, so wearing virtually no make-up; working on television up to the last newscast of the evening, in which case I will have had to touch up my make-up repeatedly throughout the day; or if I have been making a public appearance perhaps followed by a dressy evening function at which I would wear a full make-up. Never kid yourself you can skip cleansing your face late at night by using excuses such as 'I have not put any make-up on today' or 'It is so late now I may as well leave my face dirty because I'll be up again in a few hours'.

I hope you would never go to bed without brushing your teeth. Make a night cleansing routine just as automatic so that you never consider whether it is necessary or not – it is always essential.

There are five steps in night cleansing: removing make-up, cleansing the skin, toning the face, moisturizing the face, nourishing and extra-moisturizing problem areas. You may, like me, combine removing make-up with cleansing the skin but remember that they are two distinct aspects of the routine. I will go through the basic routine in detail when I have covered the other elements of the simple beauty routine.

Having thoroughly cleansed your face and neck at night you will require a less vigourous cleansing in the morning. This part of the routine depends largely on your skin type. If you have a greasy complexion then the glands below the surface will have excreted sebum during the night so you will need to cleanse the skin well. If, at the other extreme, you have dry skin you may find that you need no more than to rinse and tone the skin before moisturizing in the morning.

At night you nourish your skin, particularly any dry, lined and sensitive areas around the eyes. In the morning, moisturizing and nourishing is equally important. You are going to bare your face to the elements, and cold winds are as damaging as hot sun. You will collect grime on the skin's surface so your face needs protecting. You may be facing a day in an over-heated environment so your skin needs plenty of moisture to counteract the dehydration which will occur.

The quick morning cleanse involves removing any sweat, oil or dirt which has gathered on the skin overnight, toning the skin, moisturizing and extra-moisturizing as necessary with nourishing products. Always include moisturizing as an important part of cleansing – the two go hand in hand.

What happens during the rest of the day will determine how much attention you give your complexion between morning and night cleanses. Make-up in itself is not harmful to the skin. That is if you use the right products for your skin-type, nothing too crude or heavy, and nothing to which you are allergic. And, of course, you must remove it thoroughly at the end of each day. Make-up can assist in protecting your skin by forming a barrier against the elements and against dirt.

I am a firm believer in the fact that if you spend five minutes each night, and even less each morning, then you are helping the skin look after itself during the day. Make-up merely enhances your face. It is your skin-care routine which will finally have an impact on the look and feel of your complexion. If you look good without make-up then you'll look even better with it. If you look dreadful without it because your skin is in bad shape, then no amount of pancake and powder will give you a glowing, attractive face – more likely you will have a flat mask which is terribly unflattering. Now that you are improving your skin, you will find that your make-up lasts longer, looks better and can be applied more sparingly to allow the real, glowing you to show through.

A note on products

I hope that by now you will have realized how very important it is to have a clean and properly moisturized skin. What you purchase depends very much on your pocket. Buy the most expensive if it satisfies your ego and you like pretty matching pots on the dressing table or in the bathroom cabinet.

However, the *basic* ingredients in what you buy vary little and with the dearer products you are paying quite a lot for fragrance, packaging and advertizing. Within the purchase price you will be contributing towards research laboratories and advertizing but I've yet to be convinced that *any* product from *any* house will work miracles. It is no use spending a fortune on products and having a lousy diet, plenty of alcoholic drink, and not cleansing your skin properly.

You are probably asking yourselves what I use – the answer is a mixture. I've never gone for the dearest or the cheapest. I veer towards products which use plant extracts, partly on humanitarian grounds but also for good cosmetic reasons. Plants contain enzymes which in turn contain protein and they stimulate the processes in your skin cells, making it firmer. It's extremely difficult to do a controlled experiment on oneself. However, I had tried so many creams on my neck with little or no effectiveness that when I heard of a French plant-based product, which came highly recommended, I thought there would be no harm in making another attempt. I can say that after three months of use, I could see an improvement in my neck – the bracelets are still there but the skin is fresher and plumper. I have tried other products by the same company, and though nothing has had as dramatic an effect as the neck cream, I'm more than happy with the results.

The main points to make about products are: never be bullied into buying something you do not feel is right for you by an intimidating sales person; never believe what you read in advertisements but always try products at the counter and think about how they fit into your beauty routine and if they are correct for your skin type; do not assume that by spending less you are necessarily saving money in the long term – you may have to use so much more of a cheap product that it is financially counter-productive; neither should you assume that by spending more you are automatically going to get the best results.

Another thing to remember is that your complexion needs variety and change – do not always use exactly the same products in exactly the same way, day in and day out. For example, if you have a greasy skin and only require a light night product, you could treat yourself to a heavier night cream a few times a month.

Conversely, if you have a dry skin like mine, where I use a fairly rich night cream, once a week I either go without or use a lighter treatment.

A note on cleansing equipment

Always use the softest, most absorbent materials on your face. Remember that tissues are produced from the end product of timber – they contain fibres and can be harsh on the face. As a result, many beauticians recommend removing make-up with cotton wool but that too can be problematic. It is quite difficult to get pure cotton wool these days – it is usually mixed with viscose or some other fibre which is not as absorbent as natural cotton. Also, I find that cotton wool, unless dampened, leaves fine threads which get caught on my eye-lashes.

I always use the finest tissues – the softest available. Alternatively, if you prefer cotton wool, then I recommend cotton-wool pads which come in long packets. To avoid fine threads, always fold the pad as you use it.

If you use water in your routine and need to pat your face dry, ensure that you use either a clean face flannel, your own personal face towel, or soft tissues. Never grab the bath towel to dry your face – you will be rubbing germs and grime on to the skin you have just cleaned.

The equipment you will use most is your hands so before you start give them a thorough wash – dirty hands will merely add new grime to that you are attempting to remove.

Five-minute night cleanse

Removing eye make-up

I start my cleanse with my eyes. Assuming that you wear eye make-up you will need an appropriate eye make-up remover. The skin around the eyes is particularly sensitive so it is not wise to use the same cleanser you use to remove the rest of your make-up. A general purpose cold cream or oily cleanser is too heavy for delicate eye tissue so do not save time and money here. If you do use a heavy cream you will find yourself developing puffy eyes, and spending money in the long term trying to get rid of eye wrinkles.

There are many cleansers available for removing eye make-up – they are specially created to melt the make-up and slide it off the skin without pulling the tissue. I use waterproof mascara, and several applications, and I find that one of the new gels for removing eye make-up is best for me because it really gets rid of the mascara, and deals very well with eye liner and eye shadow.

Dot the eye make-up remover around the eye and dab it across the surface of the

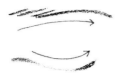

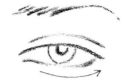

With the eye closed, start at the inner corner and stroke along the brow bone, then along the lid, to the outer corner.

With the eye open, stroke gently along starting from the inner corner, without dragging the skin.

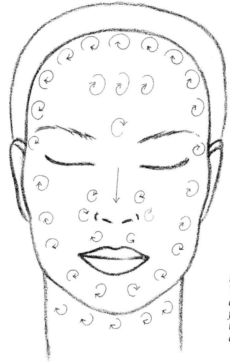

Removing eye make-up

Removing make-up
With your fingertips dot small amounts of cleanser round your face and use tiny circular massaging movements to both cleanse and improve circulation.

skin – be very gentle. Allow a few seconds for the remover to soak in. To take it off, use very, very gentle strokes. First, with the eye closed, start at the inner corner and stroke outwards under the eye. Then, again starting at the inner corner, stroke outwards and upwards across the eye-lid.

Removing make-up from the face

As you remove make-up from your face, and then cleanse and tone it, you can also give yourself a mini-massage which is helpful to the complexion. Never be rough with your skin and never just smear on a cleanser and then rub it off in a haphazard way. Instead, quickly master the correct movements shown in the diagram.

There is a wide variety of products available for removing make-up from the face. As with eye make-up removers, they are designed to melt the make-up and slide it off the surface of the skin. Soap should never be used for this since it is too harsh on the skin and not efficient in getting rid of make-up. Which product you choose will depend on your skin type and the amount of make-up you wear.

I have a sensitive skin which tends to be dry so I use a gentle liquid cleanser which is not too greasy. Basic cold cream is adequate to remove make-up and may be necessary if you wear a lot of make-up. However, if you have a greasy skin, use a gentle cleanser which will not over-stimulate the sebaceous glands and produce even more sebum.

Put a small amount of cleanser into the palm of your hand. Using the fingertips, dip into the cleanser and with circular movements work up the face, moving up-wards and outwards.

Apart from the cleansers made by the various cosmetic companies, and basic cold cream, another good product for removing make-up is pure liquid paraffin – and it is cheap enough to buy and experiment with.

Cleansing the face

Once the make-up is removed you can then clean the skin. I do this by another application of make-up remover since I find this quite adequate to clean my face. When I have been working on television, and my make-up is heavier, I may apply the remover up to three times. I use a milky cleanser specially formulated to remove make-up and cleanse the skin. However, if you remove your make-up with an oily lotion or with heavy cold cream then you should further cleanse the skin.

There are many people who do not feel that their face is clean unless they have washed it. I never wash my face, and have not done so since my teens. However, it is highly effective, particularly if you have greasy skin, but only if you use a product specially designed for facial washing. Never use ordinary soap. Soap contains deter-gents and these alter the acid/alkaline balance of the skin. Detergents remove the acid so effectively that they leave the skin alkaline. The acid on the skin's surface is important as part of its natural protective layer. Acid helps prevent bacteria and other micro-organisms from entering the skin. Using ordinary soap, you are stripping the skin of acid and allowing the entry of bacteria.

Today there are many cleansers available, including special 'soaps', which do not contain harmful detergents but which do allow you to wash your face. There are foaming cleansers, solid cleansing blocks, clay cleansers, and inexpensive, medicated creamy cleansers, all to be used with water. Whatever you choose, always rinse the face with at least fifteen splashes of clean water to remove every trace of the cleanser. In fact, if you use a cleansing cream or liquid but like the feel of water on your face, simply splash fifteen times as if you had used a substitute soap. Water is essential to the skin, so splashing the face can be highly beneficial. Ensure the water is neither too hot or too cold – it should be tepid. And never rub the face dry. Pat it dry with something absorbent and absolutely clean.

Toning the face

A toner removes any remaining traces of cleanser from the face, closes the pores, and stimulates and smoothes the skin's surface, giving a fresh, tingling feeling. Types of toners vary from those which are strong and contain alcohol – astringents – to gentler toners with no alcohol – fresheners.

I never use a toner containing alcohol – I find them far too strong for my skin and they are not generally recommended for women over thirty-five. However, many people do use astringents and find them effective in helping to prevent open pores and in removing dead skin cells from the surface of the face. If you have thicker, oily skin, then an astringent may be right for you but if an astringent has a really drying effect on your skin and makes it feel taut then abandon it.

For years I used a harsh, tingling astringent on my skin, I must admit. I believed it was correct and I could have been right since my skin was greasier then. Now I am much more gentle.

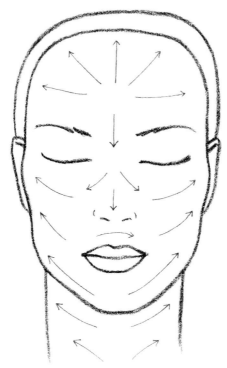

Toning
Do not rub the skin with the toner, but use gentle one-way strokes as indicated, starting with the neck.

25

Whether you are using a tissue or cotton-wool pads, dampen the material first. This will make the toner go further and add useful moisture to your face. Using a small amount of toner, start at the neck and work upwards and outwards, working up the face. Wipe down the nose and cheeks and up across the forehead. If you see signs of grime after you have applied the toner, then make a second application.

Cleansing the neck

Do not forget to cleanse your neck, along with your face, and then to tone it in the same way. You probably wear make-up on it and, together with your face and hands, it is the most exposed part of your body. Use upward stroking movements.

Moisturizing the face

Protecting and moisturizing the skin at night is as important as during the day. We spend a third of our lives in bed and the skin needs nourishing while we are asleep. The type of moisturizer you use depends on your skin type. Dry skin requires a creamy moisturizer. Greasy skin needs a lighter, fluid moisturizer. If you have combination skin you may need to use two moisturizers – a light one for greasy areas and a creamier one for dry areas. It is never advisable to use a greasy moisturizer, such as baby oil, which stays on the surface of the skin. A moisturizer carries water into the skin and provides an artificial layer of protection to assist your natural layer of sebum in protecting the skin from evaporation and dehydration.

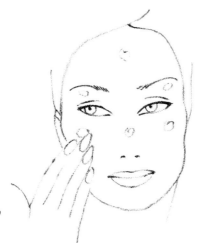

Moisturizing the face
Dab on the moisturizer, then rub in gently. Never drag or pull the skin on your face.

Eye cream

Do not use your facial moisturizer around the eyes – it is almost definitely too heavy and will cause puffiness. Eye creams are particularly gentle and should be used day and night. Dab a tiny amount around the eye, never rubbing the delicate skin, working from the outside and applying the cream above and below the eye.

There are now eye gels available, which are particularly light. I use a gel in the morning and a cream at night. Using too heavy creams around the area is one of the major causes of bags under the eyes.

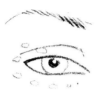

Eye cream
Dot the cream round the eye

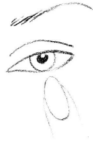

Dab gently at the skin until the cream is absorbed.

Moisturizing the neck

Again, do not forget the neck. It is one of the first areas of the body to show age – becoming crêpey, lined and wrinkled. Using gentle but lifting strokes, start at the base of the neck and work upwards using the fingertips. Then, using both hands, one after the other, stroke upwards from the base of the neck to the chin until the moisturizer has been absorbed.

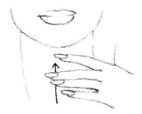

Moisturizing the neck
Apply your moisturizer with upward strokes

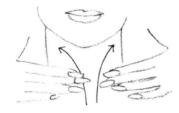

Stroke upwards with alternate hands until the moisturizer is absorbed.

Extra moisture

Enriched moisturizers, containing proteins such as collagen, are important as you get older in order to maintain the moisture level of your skin and to keep it elastic and supple. There are an enormous variety available, so seek advice. There are special anti-wrinkle creams, neck creams, night creams, firming creams and so on. It is best not to use them on the centre of your face if you have combination skin, but to use them on the forehead, cheeks, lips and, very important, the neck, in addition to your basic moisturizer.

Night creams are usually quite rich and heavy and you may find you do not require one but can merely use an enriched moisturizer night and day. I do use a night cream – a rich, corrective cream which is easily absorbed at night when my skin is no longer under the attack of extremes of temperature, make-up and general pollution.

I also use a neck cream but, again, an enriched moisturizer may be sufficient for you if your neck is not particularly lined.

Morning cleanse

Make-up removal is not necessary in the morning but if you have a greasy skin you will still need to clean it when you wake up to remove excess sebum. A quick cleanse with make-up remover (which I use) or a cleanser or wash product is usually advisable but you may only need to rinse your face in the morning.

Follow this with the same toning lotion as you use at night and then thoroughly moisturize, using a basic moisturizer and an enriched one on problem areas such as the neck. Also use your eye cream or gel beneath make-up.

Now you are ready to apply your make-up and you have completed the basic beauty routine.

Deep cleansing

I have mentioned exfoliation, a grand word to describe the shedding of old cells from the skin's surface. Regular deep cleansing is essential to help this process and help it you must. Your skin cannot benefit if you have a barrier of dirt and old cells between you and the products you choose to use. Creams and lotions will do as much good to your complexion as fertilizer would to your garden if it were piled on top of plastic sheeting rather than directly on to the soil.

Until about a decade ago, almost the only things you could buy for a good scrub of the skin were pore grains. Today there are innumerable products on sale.

Some of the more gentle products can be used daily. These generally combine mild, gritty abrasives with a cream base which you massage into the skin, leave for a few minutes and then remove – taking the dead skin cells with it. These gritty scrubs come in stronger forms to be used once or twice a week. Pore grains are similar and should be used about once a week.

You must judge carefully what you use and how often depending on the reaction of your skin. Do not overdo the process and always avoid dry and sensitive areas especially around the eyes. You may find that you need to exfoliate the central panel of the face more often than your cheeks if you have combination skin.

I use an exfoliating cream about once a week. I apply it just before getting into my bath and after washing I relax for a few minutes. I remove the cream with splashings of tepid water. And then I tone and moisturize – essential after exfoliating.

There are other methods which do not involve grains or gritty scrubs. There are brushes which can be used with your cleanser or soap-replacement. There is a buffing-pad available. You can also get small exfoliating machines which buff the skin. I have to admit I did buy one but it stands unused – I never have time to plug it in and go through the process.

In addition to regular exfoliation, you should have an occasional thorough deep cleanse using either a mask, steaming or, perhaps, a salon treatment.

Masks

I use a mask once a week when I put aside an hour for myself. I use this time for other things including my nails and perhaps giving my hair a deep conditioning. Make a beauty hour for yourself once a week. If you have a totally erratic schedule like mine then that is easier said than done.

There is an enormous range of mask (face pack or home facial) products on the market. Some form a mud-like crust on the skin, others come in the milder form of

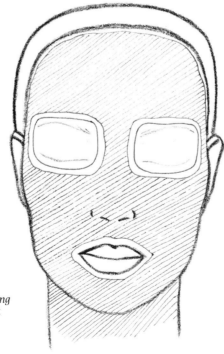

Applying a mask
Put the mask on evenly, avoiding eyes and lips, and put your feet up while it does its work with soothing pads on your eyes.

gels which peel off when dry. I find occasionally that it's satisfying, not only to the skin but also to the soul, to make your own mask. I have included some recipes for these, as well as other homemade skin-care products, at the end of this chapter.

Obviously, the oilier and coarser your skin, the stronger the mask it can take so face pack masks can be used. If you have drier, sensitive skin use peeling gel masks.

Apply the mask, usually with your fingers but with a brush if it comes in liquid form, evenly over the face. Avoid the eye area and the mouth – and do not forget your neck. Leave it on for about twenty minutes and relax as much as possible during that time. Best of all, if you can afford the time, lie down with your feet up against a wall, at an angle of forty-five degrees, and place some cotton-wool pads soaked in witch hazel over your eyes. The pads are soothing and relaxing.

Try and give yourself a mask facial on a day when you do not have to apply make-up straight away or when you can go to bed afterwards. It is rather a shame to give yourself a wonderful cleanse and then clog the face again with make-up.

Steam cleansing

An alternative to a facial mask is steam cleansing – you could use them alternately. Facial saunas can be bought which clean the skin thoroughly but a good steam – using a basin filled with steaming water and herbs – is just as effective.

Do not steam your face if you suffer from broken capilliaries – little, red, thread-like veins on the face.

You need water hot enough to give off steam but not too hot. Before adding the water, place some herbs in the bowl – preferably fresh but dried ones will do. Use about a handful of lavender, rosemary, balm, mint or camomile. Take a towel large enough to cover your head and the bowl. Place your face over the bowl and drape the towel over your head so that it covers the sides of the bowl. Hold your head there for only a couple of minutes – just time enough to allow the pores to open and absorb the aromatic vapour. Afterwards, splash with tepid water and pat the face dry with a towel. Then apply a gentle toner and moisturize.

Never overdo steaming. If you have a normal or dry skin, too much will make the skin drier, and with oily skin, steaming will over-stimulate the glands and produce unwanted sebum.

A credo to adopt for all your beauty routines is 'moderation and gentleness'. You are dealing with a delicate subject – never be rough.

Salon treatments for deep cleansing

A salon exfoliation or deep cleanse can be far more beneficial than anything you can do at home. I manage to have a 'disencrustation' about every six to eight weeks, when I visit my hairdresser who also has a small beauty salon. It is worth saving up for the occasional salon treatment and the benefit of professional advice.

There is a vast range of treatments from basic beauty masks, similar to those you can apply yourself at home, to more complex treatments involving machinery. This can all be rather daunting but your beauty therapist will tell you which treatment is best for your skin type. What may be suitable for a friend's skin may not be for you so do take advice.

I have a treatment called 'galvanic disencrustation' involving the use of an electrode. It causes the pores to relax and produces negative and positive ions which in turn produce chemical changes on the skin. Blockages, such as sebum in the pores, whiteheads and blackheads, are dissolved. Oiliness is checked and engrained skin blockages, due to insufficient skin cleansing, can be dissolved over a period of time. I am amazed at the amount of muck it removes from my face. This type of treatment is not suitable for extremely dry or mature complexions.

Other salon treatments include vacuum suction, which literally sucks waste products from the skin and massages it, causing the blood supply to increase and stimulate the sebaceous glands to give the skin a moist and supple quality. Again it is not suitable for delicate, sensitive or mature skins.

Another treatment which increases blood circulation, and so cell replacement, is one using a high frequency machine. You hold an electrode and an electric current is drawn off the surface of the skin. The electrode can be applied directly to the skin and then has a germicidal and drying effect which helps prevent spots by clearing the skin of bacteria. It also heals existing spots and blemishes, and is useful for anyone suffering from acne or greasy skin. The machine must not be used on sensitive skin or easily reddened skin with broken veins. Without actually applying the electrode directly to the skin, this treatment has the effect of relaxing the nerve endings and is useful for ageing or wrinkled skin and for skin with poor muscle tone.

Another treatment incorporating the use of electric current is the facial 'faradic machine' which produces an alternating current to increase the blood supply which contracts, and then loosens, the muscles. Again, waste products are removed and essential nutrients taken to the cells.

Paraffin wax treatment helps remove bacteria build-up and dead skin cells and also aids the acid/alkaline balance of the skin – the pH balance. This is particularly beneficial to dry, dehydrated, mature, crêpey, fine-lined and uneven textured skin.

Ozone steaming applies a jet of vapour to the skin. The ozone is produced in this method because the vapour passes over a quartz tube before reaching the face. Slight perspiration is induced and the skin becomes softened and moisturized. This aids the shedding of dead cells, helps destroy bacteria, increases blood circulation and nourishes the tissues. Other vapourizers merely spray liquid on the face under pressure – forming a thin, penetrating film which is readily absorbed into the tissues. Toners and astringents are used and their effect increased by this method.

Vibratory treatments stimulate the surface of the skin and underlying tissues, increasing the production of sebum and relaxing the tissues. Audio-sonic vibrators have a deep effect and are beneficial to sensitive, mature skin with loose tissue, and to normal, dry, and dehydrated skins. Percussion vibrators work more on the skin's surface and are beneficial to dry, dehydrated, normal and mature skins with firm contours.

These are some of the more common treatments and I hope my short descriptions will help you decide which one is right for you. I repeat, however, that you should take professional advice.

Do not ever have a salon treatment on the day you want to look your best. Make an appointment for at least five days before because the stimulation resulting from these treatments can result in small spots coming to the skin's surface. It does with me. This is merely the skin's way of throwing off the muck that was previously trapped under the tough, horny layer of dead cells. My skin looks its very best about a week after treatment.

If you cannot find the time, the money, or the salon for these treatments then merely ensure that you set aside some time occasionally for an attentive home facial, using a good mask, massaging the face, relaxing thoroughly and giving your skin a really good cleanse.

Problems

Spots

If you are unfortunate enough to suffer from spots, then you already know that there is no easy solution. Acne can become a problem at any stage in your life and if you do suffer from it then seek medical advice. If your skin occasionally breaks out, make sure you are cleansing it thoroughly and check your diet. I get spots during my periods or if I've indulged in too much rich food. Sometimes they occur when I'm overtired and, ironically, when I've had a thorough facial at the salon.

Medicated products can help but they only treat the surface of the skin, killing off bacteria there. However, the problem is usually far more deep-rooted, particularly if it is serious and widespread and you have been suffering for some time.

Basic steps can be taken to avoid spots and blemishes:

Do not use heavy creams to nourish areas where you break out. Use lighter, liquid preparations.

Avoid rich food and over-sweet indulgences such as chocolate.

Your hands carry germs, so always wash your hands thoroughly before applying skin-care products or make-up.

Stress could be a cause of spots since tension causes an over-production of sebum.

Make sure you deep cleanse regularly in order to unblock clogged pores which lead to blackheads and pimples.

Do not touch or squeeze pimples at all – unless it cannot be avoided. I must confess that I do occasionally squeeze spots but not without softening the skin first with warm water and using my index fingers covered in tissue. And only ever do this if you can see the poison – never squeeze a pimple which appears as a reddened and tender swelling since you will merely cause an abrasion on the skin, a lasting scar and you could spread the bacteria.

Use an antiseptic on the pimple – you can get creams or sticks – but apply it with a cotton-bud so that it touches only the affected area. Antiseptics are very drying.

Blackheads

Blackheads, tiny black spots on the skin, tend to occur in oily areas with enlarged pores. On combination skin this tends to be around the nose and on the chin. Thorough cleansing and toning will help, as will regular deep cleansing. Never squeeze them out – clean them out.

Whiteheads

These tiny, hard white spots often occur around the eyes and sometimes on the cheeks. Opinions differ as to how they are caused or even of what they consist. Some say they are deposits of calcium, and others maintain that they are sebum trapped in the skin. Do not attempt to remove them – they are often quite deeply embedded. Again, thorough cleansing and toning help but take time.

Broken veins

These tiny red threads on the face usually occur around the nose and on the cheeks and are caused by the capilliaries under the skin's surface expanding but then not contracting properly. When enlarged blood vessels come together they cause a reddening of the skin. The blood gets trapped in the small veins and cannot disgorge.

Alcohol is a major cause of this because it dilates blood vessels which are left with trapped blood. Spicey food can have a similar effect. Other causes include exposure to extremes of heat and cold. Do not sit too close to the fire or rinse your face in either very hot or very cold water.

A lack of elasticity in the walls of the blood vessels can help in creating broken veins and to retain elasticity a gentle tapping massage can be used. It is described in the section on facial massage in the massage chapter. Also Vitamin B aids elasticity and should be taken with Vitamin C, which helps the body retain Vitamin B. Citrus fruits are the best source of Vitamin C.

Another thing to avoid if you have broken veins is astringent and other harsh beauty treatments such as pore grains, heavy gritty scrubs and harsh soaps.

Sclerotherapy

I finally took my feet, with their broken veins, to an expert. The method which was used was sclerotherapy which applies to minor blemishes caused by broken veins on any part of the body including the face. Not all cases of broken veins are suitable for treatment and 'high colour' problems on the face may not be remedied by this method. The sclerotherapy introduces a medically approved chemical to the skin which reduces the unsightly veins and causes them to fade out like bruises. It certainly helped my feet.

Dark circles under the eyes

Lack of sleep is the basic cause so the cure is obvious. Alcohol and stress can also be a factor so try and cut down on both. The treatments for puffy eyes can help.

Puffy eyes

These are caused by fluid trapped around the eyes and will often go soon after you awake and start walking around. Obviously crying exacerbates this condition but, less obvious and equally damaging, is the use of heavy creams and cleansers around the eyes. The tissue here is extremely sensitive and the skin extremely thin.

One extra pillow can help since retained fluid can drain down whilst you sleep. You can get rid of puffiness in the early morning in several ways, and these methods also help fade dark rings under the eyes. Basically what is involved is lying down for fifteen minutes with a pad on your eyes. Use either two teabags dipped in cold water, cotton-wool pads soaked in witch hazel or two small muslin bags filled with grated potatoes.

Sun spots

Dark spots on the face and hands, and other areas of the body, are the result of too much exposure to the sun. Wear a sun-filter cream to avoid them. They can be removed, at some cost, by various processes, but undoubtedly it is best to adopt a preventative attitude and avoid exposing the skin to the sun.

Skin-care recipes

The most natural, inexpensive and pure beauty preparations are those you can make yourself. The masks take a little extra time but they are highly relaxing. When I retire I shall make all my own face and body preparations and I doubt that I'll care if I smell like a greengrocer's shop!

Toning

ROSEWATER: One of the oldest, best skin-fresheners is rosewater. It is said to have been discovered by an Arabian doctor, Avicenna, in the tenth century. He invented the means of distillation, and did his first experiments with rose petals, thus producing rosewater. When the noblemen returned from Palestine after the Crusades they brought with them rosewater, as well as the custom of offering it as washing water after a meal (necessary as they did not use cutlery!). The custom of sprinkling rosewater on the hands of guests when entering a home is still prevalent all over the Middle East as a token of welcome. Rosewater is available from most chemists but it is very easy to make your own.

GYPSY ROSEWATER: Take two handfuls of dark, scented rose petals and put them into a jar. Cover them with 1 litre (1¾ pints) of water and 250 grams (½lb) of sugar. Firmly close the top and shake vigorously. Steep this mixture for two hours, shake again then strain and store it in a cold place. To make the water fragrant, refill the jar with fresh rose petals, and repeat the shaking and steeping process until the water smells as strong as you want it.

ROSEWATER AND WITCH-HAZEL TONIC: This is probably the most famous skin tonic of all. Its fame is well deserved, mixing the fragrant rosewater with healing witch-hazel. In Brazil witch-hazel is known as the 'miraculous cure'. It is used as an antiseptic, to reduce swellings and puffiness, and as a skin tightener. All over Europe, witch-hazel has enjoyed the same popularity, and it is used a great deal in homeopathic treatments. To make this lotion simply mix ¾ cup of rosewater and ¼ cup of witch-hazel. If you have a very greasy skin you can use equal proportions of rosewater and witch-hazel.

Moisturizing and Nourishing

REJUVENATING HONEY CREAM: It is quite amazing how honey can be used for everything. It is renowned for being a natural healer; it attracts and holds moisture in the skin, ideal for counteracting dryness; and repairs and softens coarse and sensitive skin. In fact, whatever your skin type, honey can help, so use it in face masks, skin tonics, face creams, and even hair conditioners. The only trouble with honey is that it is sticky, but this next recipe avoids that.

3 tablespoons lanolin
½ tablespoon of honey
1 teaspoon lecithin
4 tablespoons warm water

Melt the oils together in a pan over a low heat. Remove from heat and slowly add the water, beating fairly fast and continuously for the first minute, and then more slowly, until it cools. This is a healing cream. Add the lecithin for extra nourishment. These quantities make about a cup of pale, creamy-coloured, firm cream or, if you leave out the water, you have about half a cup of clear, rather greasy cream. Both versions are marvellous. When you first apply it, it feels a little tacky, but it soaks in almost immediately. It is also particularly good for sallow skins as honey can bring a glow of colour to the skin, so use it daily. You do not need to refrigerate the cream; in too cold a temperature it tends to separate.

Cleansing masks

KASHMIRI FACE MASK:

> *2 tablespoons dried orange peel*
> *2 teaspoons chick-pea flour (or oatmeal)*
> *2 tablespoons cream*

Mix into a paste and apply generously all over the face and neck. After ten or fifteen minutes, when it is dry, rub it off using an upward circular motion – this abrasive action smoothes and cleans the skin. This is one of my favourites of the moment as it smells so good, and I love the thought that this recipe must have been used for thousands of years. It will suit all skin types; and is a most effective cleanser, making the skin feel smooth and satiny.

STRAWBERRY MASK: Mash up three large strawberries, apply as a mask and leave on for ten minutes. Wash off with rosewater. Strawberries are slightly acidic, containing Vitamin C. They cleanse the skin thoroughly, leaving it sparklingly clean. In fact Nero's wife, Poppaea, is said to have bathed in strawberries. If we cannot afford to do that, we can at least use this mask.

MILK MASK: One of the simplest, and probably cheapest, masks is milk. Damp some cotton wool with milk, and cleanse your face with it. The skin can benefit enormously from a quick cleanse during the day, and the full joy of this milk mask is that it is invisible, and could even be left on throughout lunch or an afternoon at the office without anyone knowing.

MIRACULOUS CLEANSING MASK:

> *1 tablespoon powdered brewer's yeast*
> *½ tablespoon yoghurt*
> *1 teaspoon lemon juice*
> *1 teaspoon orange juice*
> *1 teaspoon carrot juice*
> *1 teaspoon olive oil*

Mix thoroughly into a paste, apply and leave on for fifteen minutes. This is one of the very best cleansing masks. The brewer's yeast stimulates the flow of the blood to the skin; this nourishes it, helps healing and gives the complexion a healthy glow. (Incidentally, brewer's yeast is also marvellous for the skin when taken internally.) The yoghurt cleanses thoroughly, and the vegetable and fruit provide vitamins and minerals. This mask is suitable for all skin types, particularly if they feel and look sluggish or spotty (if your skin is very dry add more oil, and if very oily, leave it out). Use this mask in winter when one's skin has that grey, tired look: after a few applications the complexion looks alive and glowing again.

EGG YOLK MASK: When looking through beauty recipes, time and again I come across references to the miraculous properties of the egg. The yolk is full of lecithin and protein, and is very nourishing.

> *1 egg yolk*
> *1 teaspoon almond oil*

Mix together, apply and leave on the face for ten to thirty minutes. (A beautiful Belgian countess uses this every other day, and is convinced that is why her skin has remained youthful and soft.) Cream can be added to make it even more nutritious, and you could use the whole egg instead of just the yolk. Experiment to find out what most benefits your skin and wash the mask off with lukewarm water.

LEMON EGG MASK:

> *1 whole egg*
> *1 teaspoon honey*
> *1 teaspoon almond oil*

Use half a squeezed lemon as a bowl and put the yolk of an egg in it. Add a couple of drops of lemon juice and allow the mixture to stand for about half an hour. The oils from the lemon soak into the egg yolk and make this mask ideal for *greasy* skins.

AVOCADO MASK: The avocado is one of the most nutritious fruits: it contains a great number of vitamins, minerals and natural oils which can all help feed the skin.

> *2 tablespoons ripe avocado pear*
> *1 teaspoon liquid honey*
> *2 drops lemon juice*

Mash and sieve the avocado with a couple of drops of lemon juice to prevent it going black. Add the honey and mix together into a paste; apply, and leave on for as long as you can. In tropical climes this recipe is used to counteract the drying effect of the sun. It is a delicious mask, softening, moisturizing and nourishing the skin.

MAYONNAISE:

> *2 egg yolks*
> *2 tablespoons vinegar (cider vinegar preferably)*
> *¾ cup olive oil*

Crazy as it sounds, mayonnaise is an amazing beauty aid for all skin types. It has everything we need, oil to lubricate, eggs to nourish, and vinegar to retain the acid mantle. This mayonnaise can be used as a basis for masses of different fruit masks: avocados, strawberries, tomatoes, cucumbers, in fact anything you have around. If you don't have time to make your own mayonnaise, use a ready-made one, and an added egg yolk will make it almost as good as the homemade version.

CREAM AND HONEY MASK:

> *1 tablespoon double cream*
> *1 tablespoon honey*

Mix together and apply. Leave it on as long as possible then rinse off with warm water. Your skin will be left glowing and incredibly soft. A Greek woman who has a beautiful complexion recommends a mixture of milk and honey to preserve the skin. When she is cooking she has a bowl of this mixture next to her. She ties back her hair and applies the mixture to her face, with a wooden spoon, as often as possible during the time she is in the kitchen. If her skin is anything to go by, it is most certainly worth trying.

APRICOT MASK:

> *12 dried apricots*
> *10 seedless grapes*
> *Powdered milk*
> *Water*

Put apricots in a basin. Boil water and pour over until water is a few inches above the apricots. Leave to soak for 12 hours. Purée together with 10 seedless grapes and thicken with a sprinkling of powdered milk. Apply and leave for 15 minutes. Rinse off with lukewarm water.

FRUIT OR VEGETABLE JUICE MASK: For dry skin mix any fruit or vegetable juice with a beaten egg yolk and a tablespoon of honey. For oily skin mix with two teaspoons of natural yoghurt and two tablespoons of brewer's yeast.

CARROT AND TURNIP MASK: Boil the carrot and turnip and mash them into a paste. Apply the paste for 10 minutes and rinse off with milk. This mask leaves the skin feeling fresh and clean. Carrots are rich in Vitamin A which is beneficial in treating the skin and turnips (like potatoes) are marvellous cleansers.

EGG WHITE MASK: Simply spread a thin film of egg white on your face. You can use it as it is, or beat it up to a froth. Rinse off after ten to twenty minutes. This mask really tightens up the skin, ironing out wrinkles (temporarily) and leaving the skin feeling smooth and soft. It has an astringent action ideal for greasy skin. If your skin is dry add a teaspoon of oil and/or one of honey.

PARSLEY AND SPINACH TONIC MASK:

> *2 tablespoons parsley*
> *2 tablespoons spinach*

Finely chop the parsley and spinach and boil them in a cup of water for five minutes. Let this mixture cool to extract the juices fully and then strain. Use the juice as a skin tonic or thicken it with oatmeal, yoghurt or egg white depending on your skin type. Parsley cuts down the oiliness of the skin and spinach juice contains iron.

PEPPERMINT MASK:

> $\frac{1}{4}$ *teaspoon peppermint extract or oil*
> *1 egg white*
> *1 teaspoon kaolin*

Mix egg white and kaolin together into a paste and add the peppermint extract. The hot/cold effect of peppermint stimulates and tightens the skin.

DANDELION MASK: Dandelions are full of vitamins and are reputed to cure sallowness. Mash and strain two tablespoons of stewed dandelion leaves. Apply and leave for 15 minutes. Rinse off with cool water.

EGG AND YEAST MASK:

> *1 egg yolk*
> *1 tablespoon brewer's yeast*
> *1 teaspoon sunflower oil*

Mix egg, yeast and oil together to a smooth paste and apply. Leave for 15 minutes, rinse off with milk. The yeast stimulates the skin and with the addition of the egg yolk and oil is a most effective mask.

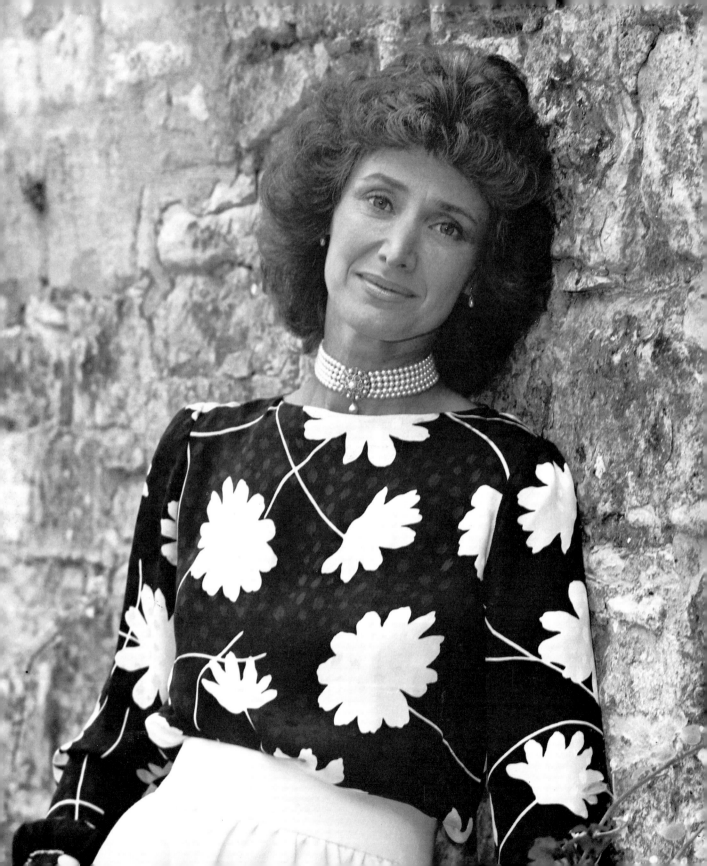

Make-up

I learnt basic make-up in my teens when I joined an amateur dramatic group. All right, the make-up is exaggerated for the stage but all the little tricks of light and shade I use to a lesser extent every day. As I have gone along my way, I've also learnt from the myriads of make-up artists with whom I've come into contact, both in the make-up room and when interviewing them in the studio. I must confess that I am rarely comfortable being made up by anyone other than myself with a few notable exceptions. It's not that I think I'm better than the professionals, just that I *know* my face instinctively. I also know what I like. For instance, I seem to have spent most of my adult life fighting off make-up girls trying to put hideously bright lipsticks on me. I didn't like them when I was younger and I certainly don't like them now – I think they are hard and ageing even on the very young.

Make-up is such a fascinating subject that one never really stops learning and experimenting – in fact it is essential that one shouldn't stop, because make-up has to be modified and adapted as you grow older regardless of the current trends.

Barbara Daly, one of the best known make-up artists in the business, was recording a series of television programmes on make-up for varying age groups. She invited me to be a guinea pig – an offer I could not refuse. She transformed me with a model look. It was most flattering but a style I could not hope to copy, nor would have the time for in my everyday life. Nevertheless it was an experience worth having and I learnt much about 'blending', particularly on the eyes. Barbara has far too busy a life to do make-ups for the masses which is unfortunate but there are establishments around the country where one can go and be made up. Large department stores frequently offer a 'make-up' when they are promoting a new product.

Applying make-up is a skill and a difficult one. One professional application is not going to teach you everything you need to know. It is best to do some experimenting at home and when you have mastered the basics, that's the time to go in for professional advice.

There are few among us who are beautiful enough, or have flawless enough complexions, not to need a little artifice. Yet it is essential to remember that make-up should enhance your face. Used with care and skill it can work wonders. Piled on to form a mask, it flattens the face and can be very ageing. It is essential to modify make-up as you grow older; if you don't it ceases to enhance. When I'm at home I wear only a touch of foundation on the most time-ravaged parts of my face – my nose and cheeks – and a dusting of powder and mascara.

Make-up is not harmful to the skin, provided you use the right products for your skin type and avoid any products to which you are allergic. In fact make-up helps protect your skin from the ravages of pollution and from extremes of heat and cold.

Make-up equipment

Brushes

For me, these are the most important aids to achieving good make-up. The good ones are not cheap but a worthy investment – they last longer and are far more effective. I now buy my brushes from artists' supplies shops; fine sable brushes used for painting and artwork. Over the years I have bought various types of brushes and packs of brushes sold by various cosmetic houses but I have never been totally satisfied with the complete range in a pack. Some tend to be too hard or the wrong thickness. Obviously it may not be necessary for you to buy all the brushes listed below but I have all eight in constant use.

2 flat, 5 mm brushes	for *eye-shadow*
1 soft, large brush	for *blusher*
1 flat, 4 mm brush	for *lips*
1 flat, 5 mm brush	for *concealing spots and under-eye shadows*
1 very fine brush	for *eyeliner*
1 soft, large brush	for *removing excess powder*
1 child's toothbrush	for *eyebrows*

Other equipment

Cotton buds	for *the removal of splodged mascara and creeping eye-shadow*
Sponges	for *applying foundation*
Puffs	*the velour kind for applying loose powder (you need at least two and they must be regularly washed)*
Pencil sharpener	

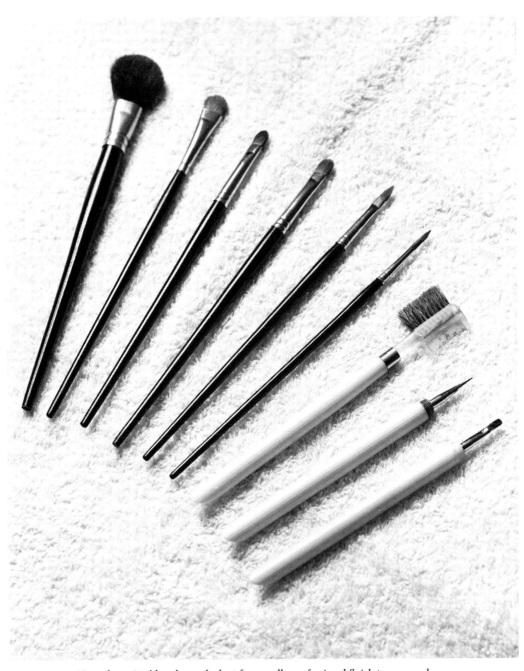

My eight artists' brushes – the best for a really professional finish to your make -up

43

What you need

Foundation

These come in different shades, of course, and varying consistencies. There are creams in jars, sticks, compressed cakes (which you apply with a dampened sponge), and liquid in bottles and tubes. I've tried them all and I favour the liquid because I find it easier to spread evenly. Make-up artists are able to use the sticks and cakes effectively but the average woman tends to be a bit heavy-handed and ends up with a mask-like look. My skin is far from perfect but I'd rather cover the blemishes with a medicated spot coverer and then put on a none-too-heavy foundation.

Most cosmetic houses offer a comprehensive selection of shades, so there should be something to suit your skin tone. Take a mirror to the daylight and have a good look at your skin to decide whether yours is light, medium, olive or dark. (Look at the skin above your wrist on the inside of you arm – the skin-tone there is more or less the same as on your face.) If you cannot decide, then see if you could persuade the sales assistant at the cosmetic counter to take you to the daylight and look. All the ghastly fluorescent light in stores makes it very difficult to truly assess colours – my make-up drawer is full of discarded nail varnish and lipstick which looked fine in the shop! And one word of warning to those of you with an oily skin – choose a foundation lighter than you think you require. You might start the day looking pale and wan but at least you won't go orange a few hours later.

If you have reasonably good and unblemished skin then you can get away with no foundation and instead use a moisturizer to the same effect for protecting the skin. You can now obtain tinted moisturizers which provide extra warmth to the skin's natural colouring. They are particularly effective in the summer.

Powder

An absolute 'must' is *loose* powder for dusting over your foundation. There's usually a choice of translucent, beige tones, slightly warmed peach tones and dark tones (though all the cosmetic houses will call them by different names). If you are unused to make-up, I would suggest that you use translucent. Although you will look pale to begin with, after about ten minutes your foundation shade will show through giving you colour enough. Buy untinted *compressed* powder for your handbag and the inevitable touching up process. If you use a strong colour, after endless nose dabbings, you end up looking clown-like. As the day progresses and you need to eradicate the shine, compact powder gives you better cover. Also, carrying around loose powder can be disastrous!

Eye-shadow

Here I come down strongly on the side of powder shadows, either loose or compressed. They are more subtle than cream shadows and, what is more important, they are more controllable and don't wear into lines on your eyelid creases. Shadow pencils are very popular at the moment but I have to admit that I simply don't get on with them. Make-up artists use them to great effect but then they are practised in their art. Try them by all means but if you're a novice, experiment with powder shadow first. What colour to buy? I may be an old stick-in-the-mud but, on the whole, I feel that shadows complementing your eye colouring are the best and you'll need three – two shades of the same colour and a light shadow for highlighting. Don't get me wrong, I simply love the mixtures of pinks, golds and peacocks on the eyes of the teenagers and cosmetic counter-assistants – they are beautiful and striking. However, for everyday wear, make-up should be unobtrusive.

So I'm still not giving you any help. I will list below, in descending order of suitability, the colours that most enhance eye colouring:

Blue eyes: *Blue, grey, sludgy green, plum, brown (if tanned)*
Blue/Grey eyes: *Blue, grey, sludgy green, plum, brown (if tanned)*
Green eyes: *Green, blue, brown, rust*
Amber eyes: *Amber, brown, rust, subtle greens*
Brown eyes: *Lucky you! Almost any colour except blue*

I would suggest that you buy your shadows individually. I have never yet used more than one colour in those 'three or six colour palettes' that most cosmetic houses sell. However a good buy, so that you can experiment whenever you wish, is one of these enormous palettes containing up to a dozen shades. They are occasionally on special offer if you buy something else and they are extremely good value. Powder shades don't go off and you've got virtually every colour you'll ever want to use. Apart from the fact that I no longer have time to go mooching round cosmetic counters trying out this and that, my days of the impulse buy are over. Recently I threw out two polythene bags full of eye-shadows, lipsticks and assorted cosmetic paraphernalia that I'd been talked into buying over the last few years.

Lipstick

Very much a matter of personal choice. I've already said my piece about dark lipsticks being hard and ageing. Go for a deep *tone* rather than a *dark* colour. I've never economized on lipsticks, always going for the better makes that are softer and full of lubrication for the lips. (Incidentally, some of the better lipsticks are so soft they need to be kept in the fridge overnight in the summer to strengthen them for a day in your handbag.)

If you're changing your lipstick, I suggest that you test the colours you're considering on your inside wrist and go off to do the rest of your shopping. A chemical reaction takes place between the acid in your skin and the lipstick and a colour change occurs. At the end of your shopping, go to the nearest 'natural' light and look again at the colour or colours before you buy. I don't think anyone needs dozens of lipsticks in their make-up drawer. One pink tone veering towards red (for those of you who like your reds) and a peach tone going to orange, with perhaps a tawny shade for darkening either in the evening. That should be enough to go with almost any colour of clothing you choose to wear.

Blusher

Again, I prefer the powder blushers but if your preference is for cream, liquid or gel remember to apply it *on top* of your foundation and *under* your powder. Never attempt to apply a cream over a powder – it won't spread evenly. The same colour of blusher can take you through the day into the evening – applied lightly for daywear and more dramatically after dark.

Fair-skinned: *a pink shade*
Olive-skinned: *a tawny shade*
Dark-skinned: *a reddish to rust shade*

Mascara

This is probably one of the most essential of all make-up aids, even if you wear precious little other make-up. Few of us have luscious lashes or even double rows like Elizabeth Taylor is reputed to possess, so a touch of artifice is a must.

Mascara comes in blocks to be used with water and a brush (and don't spit on the block! – your saliva is crawling with germs which you are then putting back onto one of the most sensitive areas of your face). The block and brush is a trifle old-fashioned these days but you can get an extremely good build-up on the lashes with repeated applications – hard to remove though! Most women tend to use the wand mascara which comes either waterproof or not. As I tend to cry easily, with emotion or laughter, and as it rains a lot in England, I favour waterproof mascara though it is more difficult to remove. These wand mascaras come with or without 'bits' – by that I mean fibres which are left on your lashes and give them the illusion of being thicker and longer. As lashes seem to wither with age, and mine are no exception, I use the variety 'with bits'. Coloured mascaras are all right for teenagers but I feel that black and brown are the most enhancing for most of us.

Eye-liner

This has been in and out of fashion like a yoyo over the last twenty years. Regardless, I have always worn it and intend to for at least another ten years or until my eyelids get too crêpey to take a line.

It normally comes in liquid form in bottles or in a compressed cake. I prefer the latter because I can control the consistency by the addition of water, not only in the case but on my eyelid. Applying eye-liner requires a steady hand and practice. If you want to try, don't experiment just before a big night out – give yourself a trial period of a few days.

Eyelash curlers

I've never really got on with these. They are difficult to use and I'm petrified that I'll pull out even one of my already thinning eyelashes. When I have used them, I've found that for the first half hour I look like a startled cat with eyelashes pointing vertically upwards and within an hour they're back to normal. Borrow some from a friend before rushing out to buy your own.

Eyelash tints

Very effective for fair-haired women since they give you darker lashes. However, you will probably still require mascara to heighten thickness and length. Do have your eyelashes tinted professionally – home applications can be dangerous.

False eyelashes

All right for a grand occasion but I wouldn't advocate wearing them constantly.

There are semi-permanent eyelashes which can be attached to your own in a salon. It's an expensive operation, you have to take extreme care with them, and as 'semi-permanent' only means about six weeks and not six years, I don't think I'd bother. So much can be done to enhance the eyes these days with the clever application of blended shadow.

Pencils

I find the use of pencils difficult. That's no reason to stop you experimenting if you want to. If you're making a purchase, do try them out on the back of your hand to ensure that they are creamy and soft – a hard, cheap pencil will pull on the delicate skin of the eyelid.

I do use a pencil *inside* my lower lids. Usually it's blue to complement my eye-shadow and sometimes, for more dramatic effect in the evening, I'll use black. If you don't normally wear eye make-up, I feel that pencil used in this way may appear a little theatrical.

Face Shape

Now let's concentrate on you. You will have to ascertain your face shape. There are six *basic* face shapes – round, square, oblong, oval, triangular and heart-shaped. You can enhance your shape with blusher, shader and highlighter. There's a super little box available from one of our most well-known chain stores – it contains highlighter, shader and two blushers which I'm sure would cater for the needs of all.

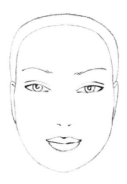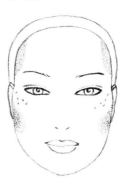

Round face
Slim down the face by using a darker foundation on the sides and a lighter tone on the central panel of the nose and cheeks. Create an illusion of more contour with shader on cheeks and highlight below eyes.

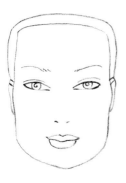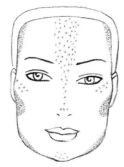

Square face
Use shading at the outer temples, outer jawline and in cheek hollows, and highlight the central panel, cheekbones and chin.

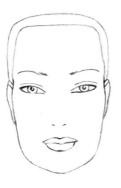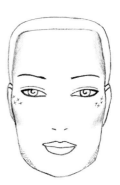

Oblong face
Shade the outer jaw to counteract a square chin, and highlight above the cheeks. Use blusher in cheek hollows, jaw-line and on temples.

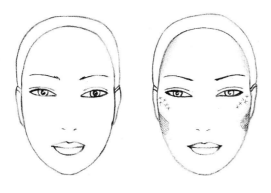

Oval face
Shade in cheek hollows and highlight cheekbones to emphasize shape. A light dusting of blusher can be used on chin and temples.

Triangular face
An angular face, so be wary of highlighters which emphasize bone structure. Use a generous amount of blusher on the lower cheeks and shaper on the chin to shorten it. A little shader on the temples will make the forehead seem less broad.

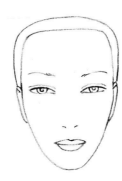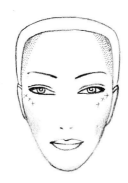

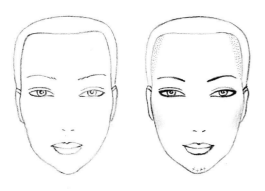

LEFT
Heart-shaped face
Many say this is the perfect shape, so just add a hint of blusher on the cheeks, highlight that small chin, and shader on the temples.

Eyes

Normal eyes

These are easy to make up. Most women want their eyes to look larger and these eyes are probably the simplest to do. You can either start with the darker shade of eye-shadow at the inner eye and blend it into the lighter shade and then to the highlighter. Or you can do as I have done and accentuate the crease below the brow with a colour such as brown and blend it outwards towards the highlighter. On the lid I usually wear blue and I blend both blue and brown under the lid.

Almond eyes

Almond-shaped eyes are most attractive and usually the possessor of a pair wishes to accentuate the shape. This is done by keeping the darker shadow to the outer corners of the eyes and taking it under the bottom lashes. You can use highlighter just under the outer edge of the brow if you wish.

Close-set eyes

Avoid any darkness near the nose. Create an illusion with highlighter or a mix of highlighter and the merest touch of shadow near the nose and gradually darken the shadow as you come out to the outer corner, extending well beyond the eye and down under the bottom lid but never further than the centre of the eye.

Deep set eyes

These are difficult eyes to deal with, but not impossible. Because the eye is deep-set and the browbone prominent, a shadow is cast over your eyes. Choose a light shade and use it over the entire lid, lightening it as you move upwards and blending it over the browbone until it fades away.

Eyes too wide apart

Obviously the reverse of the close-set eyes and the reverse treatment. Here you take your dark shadow into the inner corner of the eyes near the nose and gradually lighten as you come out to the outer corner. If you trim your eyebrows, never trim them too far apart at the centre.

Protruding eyes

Unfortunately, you are stuck with dark strong shadows for these particular eyes, blending upwards and outwards until it fades away. Just a touch of light shadow at the innermost corner of the eyes.

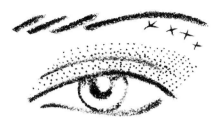

Normal eyes

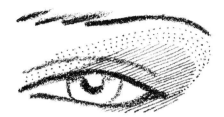

Almond eyes

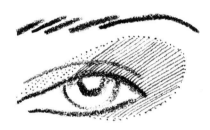

Close-set eyes

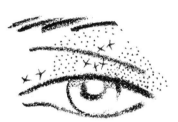

Deep-set eyes

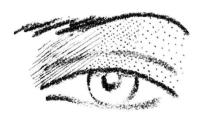

Wide-apart eyes

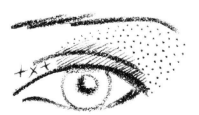

Protruding eyes

Round eyes

These can be small or large but in either case, you will probably want to elongate them into more of an almond shape. Highlight the inner corner and centre of the lid, blending in shadow between the highlights. Then apply shadow fairly heavily at outer corners taking it upwards and out towards the brow. Never take the colour beneath the lower lid – this makes the eye look even more round.

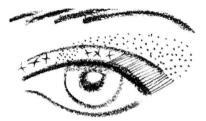

Round eyes

Lips

Lips are really not as easy to rectify as eyes. Yes, you can take your lipstick over your lipline if they are thin, below if they are too fulsome, but frankly, it always shows and I don't think it's particularly becoming. I would suggest a simple expedient. If your lips are bigger than you would like, then steer clear of harsh colours and frosted or glossy products – go for subdued shades.

If your lips are too thin, work in the reverse, *do go* for bright colours and lip gloss. And if you have one lip bigger than the other, even them up by applying the same colour to both lips and darkening the larger lip with a deeper shade of lipstick, a brownish shade – it usually blends in well with most colours. I tend to wear a peach-coloured lipstick most of the time and the quickest way to dramatize it for evening wear is just to add a coat of brown.

Many make-up artists advocate the use of a pencilled outline to the lips. I think this is fine for evening and special occasions but a little bit harsh for everyday wear. Never forget that make-up is meant to enhance the *natural* you, not create a mask.

If you are outdoors in either hot or cold weather, it's always advisable to wear lipstick because it acts as a protection from both extremes. I find that when I'm home for a few days and forget to put on lipstick, my lips very quickly get chapped. If you don't want to wear lipstick then do put on a protective coating of lip-salve.

If you find that your lipstick has a tendency to weep (run into the little lines that start to appear round the mouth) then try blotting it after application, add a fine dusting of loose powder, blot again and then apply more lipstick with your lip brush.

Teeth

What, you may ask, are teeth doing in a chapter devoted to make-up. Well they are part of your face and they are also, sadly, one of the most neglected parts of both men's and women's anatomy. I'm not suggesting that you all rush out, spend a fortune and get a mouth full of tombstones like those possessed by so many American stars. But I cannot see the point of devoting time, energy and money to improving your skin, applying enhancing make-up and then smiling to reveal ugly teeth. Decaying teeth, heavily discoloured teeth, bad gums and gaps left by missing teeth can be dealt with by your dentist provided you visit him or her regularly. Do read the section on teeth in chapter four.

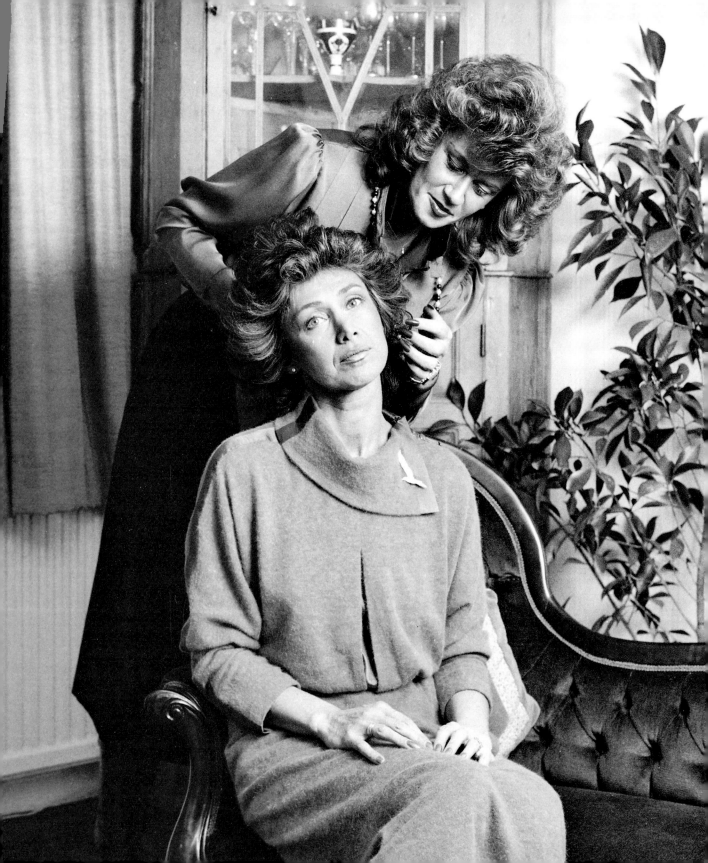

Hair

'Woman's crowning glory' – and one of her biggest headaches. Why are we so rarely satisfied with what nature gave us? I don't know – I've been just as dissatisfied as everyone else in my time. If it's straight we want it curly, and if curly we spend pounds straightening it. It's dark, we want to be blonde, it's fair and we aim for the Cleopatra look. I've tinted my hair for half my life so far – I've been chestnut, the blonde side of brown and for the most part of my adult life 'blue-black'. I am now, with just the merest help from my hairdresser, natural and greying and wondering why I ever spent so much time and money trying to be what I wasn't. I did enjoy *most* of it, particularly the dramatic black. I've had long hair which I've worn in a severe pleat, in a ridiculous beehive (all the rage at the time) and loose. I've had very, very short hair worn in an urchin cut. Actually, it's all been fun but if I were allowed to change my hair at the wave of a wand I'd ask for very dark brown, long and curly locks.

However, I'm me, and you're you, and when my hairdresser, who is also a friend, suggested that I was not going to see twenty-five again and there really was a lot of grey and shouldn't I consider toning it down a bit – I acquiesced. My hair, as I wear it now, is hard work. And don't let anyone fool you – very few women have naturally luscious locks which require no attention. Even if you have the money, I doubt that many of us have the time to visit the hairdresser three times a week. I used to enjoy a visit to the salon but for many years now I've begrudged the hours sitting around with bedraggled locks when there is so much more that I want to be getting on with. I go about once in six to eight weeks for a trim, a perm or a few perm curlers on the straighter bits (if my current style is curly), and a re-style if my hairdresser has decided to change my image.

Yes, I do more or less hand my head over to her. She's tended to my locks – black, brown, piebald, curly and straight, long and short – for fourteen years now. I have tried various other stylists from time to time but without any real success. A hairdresser really has to know your hair to be of any value to you and the odd visit doesn't give you or them a real chance. Anyway, rather like my make-up, I have an instinct for what is right for me and usually know by the way a stylist initially approaches my crowning glory whether the relationship is going to work – nine times out of ten it doesn't.

The main reasons for which I've remained loyal to my hairdresser are:

COURSES: Although she has become a highly successful businesswoman with, at one time, ten salons to her and her partner's credit, she never stops going herself and sending her staff on courses for colouring, cutting, perming and anything else new.

INDIVIDUALISM: She assesses each client's face-shape and build and she will talk you out of a style if she knows it won't suit you, or is inappropriate for your particular hair texture. A cautionary tale – many years ago, one of her male partners cut my hair and despite my protestations that I was sure it would be too severe for me, and more importantly, would look wrong on television, he proceeded merrily along his way giving me the same cut that he'd already given dozens of clients in that week. I was right and the switchboard at HTV in Bristol was jammed with viewers protesting at the 'hard' look. The audience gets very attached to us and they are not backward in coming out with criticisms. If I listened to them all, or tried to please everyone, I would have an impossible task, but on this occasion they all made, with one voice, the same criticism – it was *too severe*.

MAINTENANCE: She gives me styles which she knows I can manage – sometimes with more effort than others – for the periods in between visits, and for me that's weeks not days!

How to go about choosing your hairdresser

You will probably go to a salon that a friend has recommended. A first visit to a salon is like a lucky dip – you'll always come out with something but it may not be what you want. Here are a few basic ground rules.

INITIAL APPOINTMENT: Whether made by telephone or in person, tell the receptionist that you are a *new* client and you would like to book an appointment with the person who is best at doing whatever your particular hair happens to be – long, straight, short, curly, permed etc. The word 'new' should trigger off a response: possible future custom, must create a good impression, who is best for that particular kind of hair. If you have to wait for a day or two for an appointment, then *wait*. Try and book for a plain shampoo and set so that you can assess the situation before you get involved in heavy expenditure with new styling, tinting or perming. Some

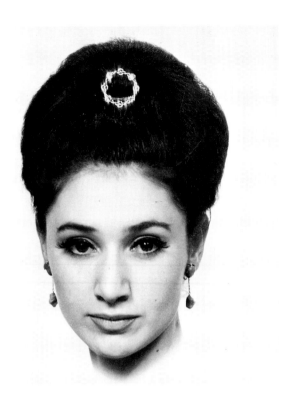

LEFT
Some of my hairstyles over the years –
this was when I was twenty.

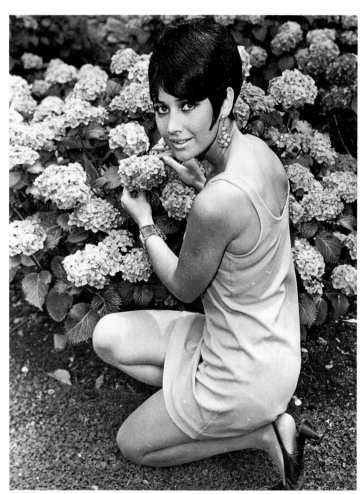

RIGHT
In 1967 I was a typical dolly-bird – pale
lipstick, black eye-liner and a sculptured
hairstyle to go with the inevitable mini.

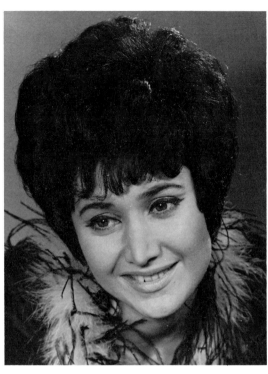

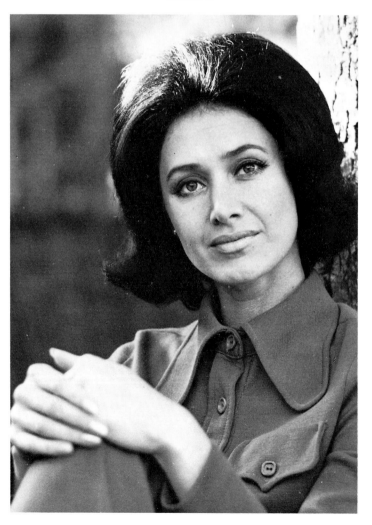

LEFT
In 1971 my hair was still black, but getting longer.

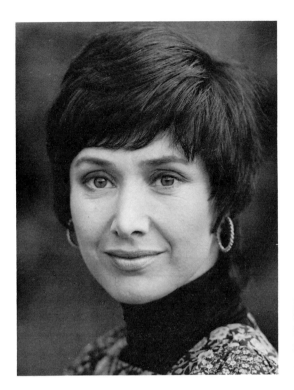

Shorn again in 1976 – a simple style that was no trouble to look after.

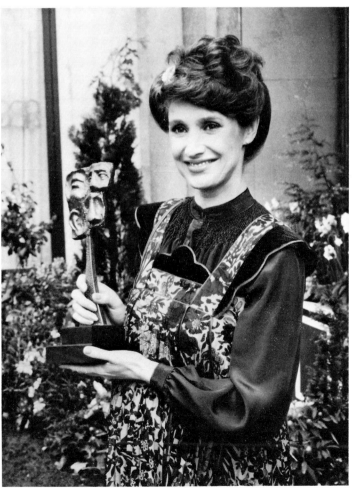

In 1981 I received the Newscaster of the Year Award – I had my longer hair up (and I was eight months pregnant).

salons don't like to accept a client unless they can do a re-style but you might be able to compromise on a trim – a regular necessity and nothing too drastic.

DIPLOMAS: I used to think that they were just there to paper the wall – they're not. They are an indication that the owner is keeping up with the times, employing staff who are qualified and is sending them on courses – provided that they aren't years out of date!

WAITING: It does seem to be traditional to be kept waiting around in the salon and a short wait is acceptable – perhaps five minutes with your hair wet while waiting for the next stage. But, if you're kept waiting too long, ask to see the manager. Don't be afraid to speak up; if there's a genuine reason, like a stylist having gone sick and others having to cover, that's forgivable but *overbooking* isn't.

CLEANLINESS: There is no excuse for hair, pins, towels and other paraphernalia to be left lying around a salon. If the management is stinting on juniors to clear up, then they're penny pinching in other ways too – using inferior shampoos, conditioners and perm lotions. Heated rollers do discolour with constant use, but they should always be clean.

When you have chosen your hairdresser, and let's hope your choice is a good one, do be guided by him or her. If you are told that the style you've picked is not suitable for your hair texture, ask what you can have that will approximate to your choice. Robert Burns wrote 'Oh, for the gift that God could gie us, to see ourselves as others see us.' It's very easy to get into a rut over style and colour of hair, particularly the latter. The rich chestnut you affected in your youth may not be so becoming as you grow older and your skin tones change – take the advice of the colourist.

Although hairdressers can do a great deal, they need a decent head of hair on which to work. All right, hair varies enormously but we can all enhance what we've got by paying attention to nutrition and making sure we get enough of the vitamins and minerals essential to beautiful hair. Most of what we need is obtained through a healthy diet but if your hair is particularly lack-lustre some extra vitamin B and E will help, as will the minerals iron (check with your doctor if you think you need iron pills) and zinc which can be found in shellfish, sunflower seeds and brewer's yeast.

Caring for your hair

The hair that the man in your life caresses is actually dead but it still needs tender loving care and attention. The living hair is the hair you don't see, embedded in its own follicle in the scalp. The follicle is fed by the papilla which is in turn nourished by capillaries that transmit nutrients. The nutrients are found in the blood – therefore good blood circulation on the scalp is important.

The outer part of your hair has layers, like a pine cone. If the layers are flat then your hair is shiny but if they are raised for any reason light doesn't reflect so easily – resulting in duller hair. My own hair, when left as nature intended, is extremely shiny. However, when it's permed, that smooth cuticle on the hair is twisted out of the norm – result, not nearly as shiny. The price you pay for artificial curls is less gloss.

Shampooing

Oh dear! The vexed question of shampooing. The argument has raged for decades against too much shampooing – it dries out the natural oils in normal hair, it overstimulates greasy hair. When my hair was short, I washed it every day for six years with no ill effects at all – but I do have strong hair and I did use a good mild shampoo. Now my hair is longer and drier because it is permed. I shampoo it twice a week. Whatever your hair type, you should wash it at least once a week. Brush or comb it through first to get rid of dirt and hair-spray if you use it, and any tangles

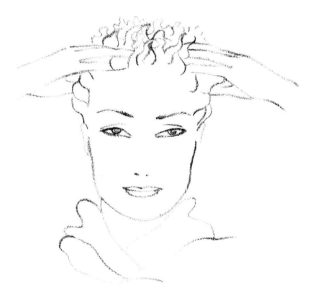

Shampooing
Use the fingertips to give the scalp a good massage at the same time.

there might be. You should never brush your hair harshly when it is wet – hair stretches when wet and any further stretching with a brush is damaging. If your hair is long, comb it gently, starting at the ends, combing through a few inches of length at a time. If you don't have a shower, under which you can wash hair, I strongly recommend that you buy a shower attachment from your chemist – they are not expensive, last for years, and do a far better job of rinsing your hair than a 'sink and saucepan' job.

Don't buy any old bottle of detergent shampoo. Choose the correct shampoo for your hair type – normal, dry or oily. Change your make of shampoo every few months – alternate your favourites, three months on and three months off. Hair, like skin, gets used to a product and ceases to benefit from it. If your hair is oily, every once in a while switch to a normal shampoo for a few washes.

On most shampoo bottles, the instructions suggest that you wash twice but if your hair is fine or you wash it frequently, then one wash is quite adequate. And don't forget the value of total rinsing – rinse and rinse again until your hair squeaks (a trifle more difficult on permed hair but when the perm has settled down, your hair will squeak again). When you are shampooing, take the opportunity to massage the scalp – it increases circulation.

Conditioning

There are deeply penetrating conditioners, more like treatments and sometimes in the form of wax and called 'masks', which are for use about once a month. I usually have one of these at the hairdressers – it's easier for the junior to section my hair and apply the stuff and I'm all for an easy life. If you don't play around with your hair – colouring, tinting, perming etc. – then it's unlikely you'll need a conditioning treatment, but they can never do any harm.

You can give yourself a deep treatment with almond oil or olive oil. Wash and dry your hair, then massage the oil liberally onto your scalp and down the hair, paying particular attention to the hair ends. Comb through, cover with a shower cap and leave overnight. Very thorough washing is needed in the morning.

The ordinary conditioner, which can be used after every shampoo if required, should be chosen for your particular *hair type*. These products do little more than coat the hair, but they do make it easier to comb and more manageable. Although a conditioner is not a deep treatment, I do like to leave it on for about five minutes. Rather than walk round the house with a wet head, I wash my hair just before a bath, apply the conditioner, get into the tub, bathe, do a few simple exercises and then rinse my hair – that means it has been on for about five minutes. Don't forget to wash your brush and comb every time you shampoo your hair – there's no point in putting lask week's dirt back into clean hair!

Drying

If you possess wonderful hair that falls just as you want it, and you have the time, allow it to dry naturally. The other ninety-nine per cent of us probably need to use a hair-drier. However, do blot off most of the water with a towel first or hair-drying will take forever. I wash my hair in the morning, prior to my television appearances, and wrapping the towel round my head in a turban, go and have breakfast. The towel 'blots' off a great deal of the moisture and there's been no hard rubbing of the hair and scalp.

If you require a setting lotion, mousse or gel, apply it while the hair is still damp – it spreads more easily. Never use the hair-drier on 'hot' for more than a couple of minutes. Turn down the setting and complete the drying process. Don't hold the drier too near the hair and do try and avoid the heat on your face. I always apply

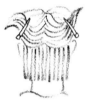

Blow-drying for medium to long hair
Make a centre-back parting and clip hair out of the way.

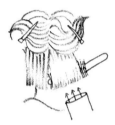

Brush up under one side of lower back hair, lift and blow-dry into shape.

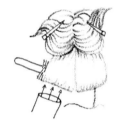

Do the same on the other side.

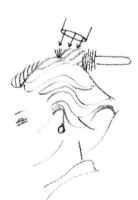

Unclip one side of upper back hair, curl round brush and dry.

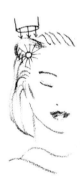

Work on small sections of hair on the sides.
Follow the same routine for the sides as for the back, always lifting the hair as you blow-dry.

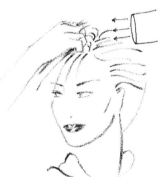
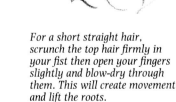

For a short straight hair, scrunch the top hair firmly in your fist then open your fingers slightly and blow-dry through them. This will create movement and lift the roots.

63

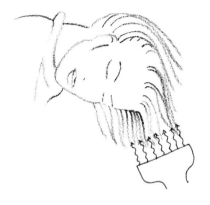

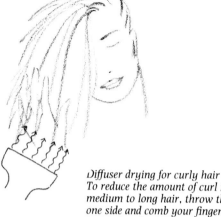

Diffuser drying for wavy hair
Throw the head forward and aim the diffuser
upwards. Move the head from side and side
and run your fingers through the hair as your
dry. This will give extra body and allow full
freedom to a natural wave.

Diffuser drying for curly hair
To reduce the amount of curl in
medium to long hair, throw the hair to
one side and comb your fingers through
it. Aiming the diffuser just above your
fingers, dry the hair as it is being
gently pulled straight. Keep changing
the position of your head so that you
don't overdry one section before going
on to another.

a moisturizer to my face before hair-drying – it acts as a barrier to the heat. I have a 'diffuser' on the end of my hair-drier – excellent for naturally curly or permed hair – about 8 inches in diameter, almost conical in shape with large holes. The hot air from the drier is then diffused through these holes instead of being concentrated on one small part of the head.

LONG HAIR: Take the bulk of the hair to the top of the head and secure with combs or grips. Using a brush to hold the hair, dry at the nape of neck and work upwards in sections. Gradually release more sections of hair from the crown, finishing at the front. Always dry the under layers first. You will discover that not only do you dry your hair quicker than trying to dry the whole lot together, but the hair is more manageable and can be coaxed under or flicked out as you go. If you want some lift in your hair, then literally lift it and dry from the roots outwards. If you are trying to overcome a natural wave, then you need to grip the hair with your brush and hold it downwards as you play the dryer over the hair, starting at the roots again.

It is not the easiest thing in the world to hold a brush correctly and use a drier in the other hand. I learned by watching the hairdresser and suggest you do the same. I can never get the back of my hair to lie as well as it does in the salon, but then I haven't got five foot arms with which to stretch my hair above my head – never mind, the rest is all right and when you have to look after your own hair, you learn quickly enough.

Wavy setting for long hair
Flexible hair-shapers are quite new, and they give you lovely soft waves. You can also use rags or strong tissues rolled into tubes to make the same effect. Although the style lasts longer if both twisted and wound, as shown below, I find it equally effective if you just wind it round the hair-shapers.

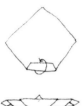

Roll tissues crosswise into tubes.

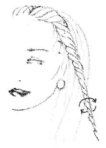

Start with a generous section of hair from the front. Hold it at the bottom and twist it along its length.

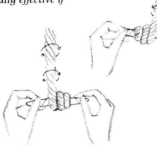

Wind it round the tube in the same direction as that in which it was twisted.

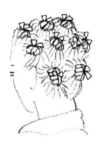

When the whole length of hair has been wound up, tie the ends of the tube together. Continue in the same way with the rest of your hair.

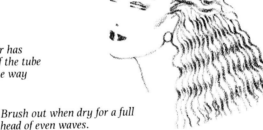

Brush out when dry for a full head of even waves.

SHORT HAIR: Deal with as for long hair – commencing at the back of the neck and working upwards in sections, finishing at the front.

PERMED HAIR: If it is permed so as to give you curls all over, let it dry naturally if you have the time, running your fingers or an afro-comb through it occasionally. If you use a hair-drier, a diffuser is excellent. If you haven't got one, then play the hair-drier gently all over the head again and again, don't play concentrated heat on one place at a time. When dry, set with rollers or heated rollers.

Hair appliances

BRUSHES AND COMBS: Never buy metal combs and don't buy a cheap brush. Bristle brushes are all very well if your hair is fine but I found that they never really gave me the feeling that I'd brushed my hair. Synthetic and combination brushes are perfectly acceptable these days as long as the 'bristles' are rounded or have 'cushion' tips. Round brushes, made with a combination of bristle and synthetic materials, grip the hair very well when you are blow-drying. Always keep brushes and combs scrupulously clean.

HEATED APPLIANCES: There are so very many heated hair appliances on the market these days that, with a little bit of practice, there's no excuse for any woman not being able to put a bit of bounce into her hair between visits to the hairdresser. *But heat is damaging to the hair and all these hair aids should be used with caution.* I'm a fine one to talk – I need to use my heated rollers practically every day of my life. When I'm not appearing on television, I'm attending conferences, seminars and the like, so that my hair always has to look as good as I can possibly get it. That's another reason for my infrequent visits to the hair salon, I simply don't have the time, and who's going to do my hair at 7.30 am so that I can appear in good order to start work at 9.00 am! I do, however, amply compensate for the drying with conditioners, treatments and trims for the split ends.

HEATED ROLLERS: These have been around for a couple of decades now and they've been improving all the time. The latest on the market are rollers covered in a kind of velour which grips, and has none of the little spikes to break, the hair. I would strongly recommend that when your current set gives up the ghost, you purchase the covered variety. Until then, if you have to use them frequently, it's a good idea to cover the spikes with strips of tissue wound around the roller.

Putting in the rollers is an art – which it has taken me years to perfect, I might add. Again, watch how your hairdresser does it. The best thing when putting rollers, heated or ordinary, is to remember that you use big rollers and larger sections of hair for a loose set, and small rollers and smaller sections for a tighter, more curly

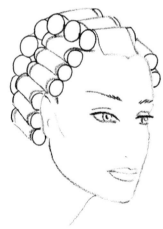

Heated rollers
Unless you put your rollers in correctly the finished effect will be untidy. Don't skimp on rollers – take small sections of hair every time, lift up at right-angles to your head, roll down to the roots and pin securely. As soon as the last one is in, the first should be ready to come out.

set. For most styles, take the hair vertically from the head, always difficult at the back, and roll tightly. Putting in the pin can sometimes present difficulties. If the pin won't hold the roller firmly, take it out and try putting it in diagonally. Don't give up with the pinning – if you leave it loose and floppy, the curl won't be as good and the roller will eventually drop out. Take time over putting in your rollers and think which way you want your hair to sit. At the moment I'm wearing my hair flicked backwards, so I pull the hair forward and then wind it, giving extra bounce at the roots.

HEATED COMBS: Used in almost the same way as a roller. Take the section you wish to deal with and run the heated comb through the hair a few times as if you were combing it, then roll the hair round and hold the comb in the hair for a minute or two. I see the heated comb as a touch-up piece of equipment for it would take a very long time to do the whole head with one unless your hair is very short.

The best equipment I've ever purchased is a cordless heated curling comb – it doesn't have to be plugged in anywhere and works off gas. Used according to the instructions it is perfectly safe. I've even touched-up my hair in the car on the way to a function – I hasten to add when I was not driving. Heated afro combs are a recent development – used as you do the non-heated variety – but obviously capable of helping dry the hair quicker. And they too are powered by gas – so take them anywhere.

BRUSHING OUT: Don't be frightened of vigorously brushing your hair when you take out rollers – if you don't you'll get gaps and regimented lines of curls. Brush your hair against the direction in which you put the rollers, bend head forward towards the chest and brush through from nape of neck, throw head back, brush through again and then start to mould your hair into the style you want. I have a 'vent' brush – with widely set apart teeth, cushioned on the tips – which separates the hair and somehow creates an illusion of you having more hair.

Hair-spray

These days it is regarded as a trifle out of date. If your hair is cut well enough and set the right way you shouldn't need spray. I keep a can in the house for difficult days. If you use it, don't economize – buy the best you can afford. Cheap hair-sprays form a build-up on the hair rather like a fine layer of glue – this attracts the dirt and is much more difficult to wash out. Always hold the spray well away from the head.

Colouring your hair

If you want to colour your hair at home, there's nothing that can go drastically wrong with a 'rinse' but I would leave 'tints' to the expert. If you're considering a colour change and aren't sure about it, then try a rinse – if you've made a mistake it will disappear after about half a dozen shampoos and no harm is done. Buy a good brand – there will usually be a table of suggestions for altering colour – and always follow the instructions carefully. A tint is in fact permanent except that, as your hair grows, the regrowth will be your original colour and you will need to 'touch-up' every six weeks at least. Bleaching, streaking, hi- and low-lights – do leave to the hairdresser.

Perming

I know it's not cheap but I really would leave this to the salon. A good perm will last you eight to twelve weeks, providing you have it trimmed a couple of times and slightly restyled to accommodate the hair growth and looser curl. Perming these days is a much more gentle process than it used to be – still as time consuming I'm afraid – but you can run your fingers through the curls when it's done. Do you remember when your hair felt like a piece of old tow-rope? There is a very quick salon perm available which is done in a matter of minutes but it is really only appropriate for fine and virgin hair – by that I mean tresses that have not been previously messed around by perming, tinting or bleaching. For every head, the first perm is always the best. After that you're curling on curl and the effect is never quite as brilliant again.

Choosing your style

What a difficult decision. What you want and what you end up with are very often two entirely different things. I loved, along with half the nation, the hairstyle worn by the Princess of Wales around the time of her wedding and afterwards. I know, deceptively simple though it looked, it was indeed a style that required the right consistency of hair, an ace cut, and a great deal of grooming. I wonder how many women tried to imitate 'the look' and failed miserably, with the sides flopping forwards within an hour or two of a set. This is the problem, you must choose a style that suits you and is right for your texture of hair. If you're not sure, then ask your hairdresser for advice and if what he or she suggests is not quite what you want then compromise and go for something in between – I must admit that many hairdressers do go over the top. And a golden rule: remember that you must *maintain* your hair in between salon visits, so go for something you know you can manage, not something that will look lousy after a day or two. This is, as mentioned before, one reason why I like my hairdresser – she gives me styles that I can manage. For a special occasion, of course, you can go a little wild and glamorous.

HAIR TEXTURE: When choosing a style some other factors have to be taken into account apart from the shape of face – texture, run and direction of growth, hair line, natural fall of the hair and the crown. Hair growing around the crown of your head very often has a will of its own – some people have double crowns and double trouble. The hair only wants to go in one direction and I'm afraid you have to follow the will of your hair, and adapt your style to fit in with the stubborn crown. With all these factors to consider you really have to depend on the advice of your hairdresser as to what is best suited to your face shape.

You can take along a picture of the style you require. Often that gorgeous style has been achieved by a certain amount of trickery. You might find that a model with more hair than she knows what to do with has very often brushed it all to the front for the photograph and there's hardly any at the back – that's fine for a photographic session but not for real life. Your hairdresser can do his or her best to approximate to the picture you've produced but unless your own hair is exactly the same texture you're not going to be one hundred per cent pleased with the result.

Don't ever change your hairstyle on the day of a big occasion, nor the colour. Many years ago I was experimenting with my hair. I decided to have a go at a chestnut hue. The junior left it on too long so that instead of looking good for the occasion I was acutely embarrassed by my flaming red hair (before the days of punk and Marti Caine). A new style also needs time to settle – two to four weeks.

Even with a straightforward shampoo and set or blow dry, I find the best course of action is to have my hair done the day before an 'occasion' and then have a comb out on the day itself.

Greying

Remember that the style you had at twenty is not going to be appropriate at forty. Also, how very boring it is to retain the same old style forever and a day. Remember that the colour you have used in your twenties is not going to be so flattering when you are older. Your skin ages, gets more sallow and wrinkles and as this process is taking place so too does your hair change. It loses pigment, becomes greyer and faded. But it does complement your skin.

I'm not suggesting that you have to go grey completely naturally if you find it unattractive but very often grey hair can be far more flattering. I know that I could no longer take my dyed black hair that was so effective and flattering ten years ago. My sister and I badgered our mother for years to stop dyeing her hair. We finally won the day – she looked prettier and younger than she had done with tinted hair.

One of my most attractive friends went grey at fifteen and it's never bothered her – I can't imagine her with anything else. Some of us, me included, are given the rather indeterminate sort of 'pepper and salt' grey hair but this can always be lifted with a water rinse – not pink or blue – to take away the yellowness.

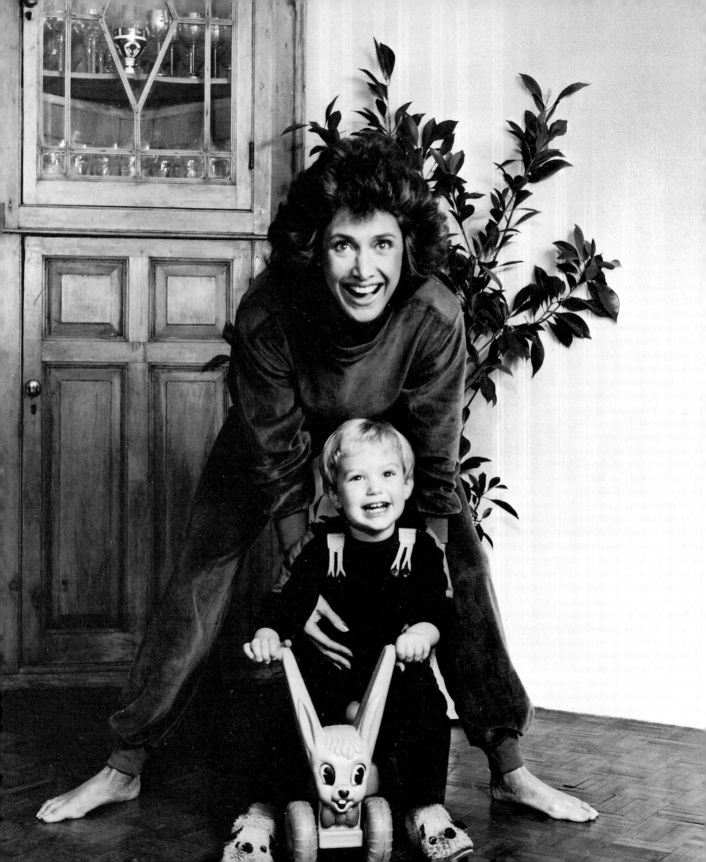

Diet and Health

The mirror test helped you assess how to change your looks and style. An assessment of your eating habits is even more important. Your general well-being, physical and mental health, body, complexion and hair condition and your weight are all determined to a great extent by your diet. Take some time to note down precisely what you have eaten, say, over the last three days and at what times you ate and in what situations. Include everything you drank as well, from water to wine. Were the vegetables fresh, frozen or canned? Was it sliced white bread or wholemeal? If you cannot remember, then over the next three days note it down after each meal, snack and drink.

The present near obsession in the western world with healthy eating has given us a barrage of information, diets, wonder discoveries, scares and strictures. It has also, with the associated interests in keeping fit and giving up smoking, cut down the number of people who die from heart conditions and other major killers. If you want to feel good, look great and get the most out of life, you *know* it makes sense to eat sensibly.

I am not an expert on nutrition but, like most of you, the recipient of endless advice and information on healthy eating. I do not intend to dictate what you eat or provide a fail-safe formula to eating well. Instead I want to help you help yourself to eat well – and to help your family.

You have heard it many times before, but what you must maintain is a balanced diet of protein, carbohydrates and fat – yes, even fat!

The reason we need a balanced diet is that our body requires to be supplied with vitamins and minerals found across the total range of protein, fat and carbohydrate foods.

PROTEIN is found in meat, fish, cheese, eggs, milk, cereals and nuts. It is essential for body growth. But it is high in calories and much of protein-rich food is high in fat and should not be eaten in *large* quantities. We probably eat far more protein than we need. If your main course was meat, then don't finish off your meal with cheese. You've already got the protein you need. If you want to gorge on cheese then have a cheese omelette for your main meal – you do not have to have meat every day. You do need protein and you can get that from several sources. I eat very little meat, preferring fish, and I'm healthy enough.

CARBOHYDRATES are in pastries, puddings, sugar, of course, and bread and cereals. These foods are low on nutrients but they do break down in the body to form glucose which is necessary to provide energy. Potatoes were long advised against as being starchy and high in carbohydrate. When not doused in cooking oil or butter, they are very good for you, especially when eaten with skins on. I started eating potatoes with their skins on years ago because I was too lazy to peel them – I was delighted to discover I'd been doing myself a favour! They contained essential vitamins and minerals.

So too does the right kind of bread – by that I mean wholemeal and wholegrain breads which also provide essential roughage. During the bread strike a few years ago, people had to eat what they could get. Many were forced to eat 'proper' bread and having tasted that didn't return to the packaged 'blotting paper' variety. Do wean yourself off white bread – make your house a 'brown' house. Wholemeal pastas, spaghetti, macaroni and brown rice are far more tasty once you get used to them, and far better for you.

FATS are found in butter, margarine, milk, cheese, vegetable oils and meat. Do cut the fat off your meat before you consume it – it does you no good at all. It makes me heave to even consider dipping into a piece of unadulterated fat. Fats do provide energy but they are very high in calories. Cholesterol is a word you've probably come across – it's cholesterol in the blood which contributes to diseases affecting the heart and circulation. So even if you're not slimming, tread warily with this group. At present our fat intake (as a nation) is some ten to twenty per cent more than is needed for a balanced diet. So very simply, if you drink a lot of milk, then don't also consume a great deal of cheese – one or the other or preferably a *little* of each. All foods in *moderation*.

ROUGHAGE: roughage and fibre, roughly the same things, have been much in the news since the advent of high-fibre diets. You need roughage to scour out your intestines and bowel. Diverticulitis is an illness which is on the increase – it's caused where soggy foodstuffs have been caught up in the multitudinous crevices along the intestine, rather like plaque building up on the teeth. The food sits there and rots – ugh! The stomach gets distended and it is extremely uncomfortable. So think 'brown' and eat wholemeal bread, wholemeal pasta and so on. Fresh vegetables, beans (including tinned baked beans – though they also contain a lot of sugar), and things such as potatoes cooked in their skins also provide roughage.

Vitamins

Vitamins act like a catalyst in chemistry, triggering off a reaction which enables the body to make use of other nutrients. The B vitamins and Vitamin C are water soluble

Make-up merely enhances your face. It is here in the bathroom that you must begin with a thorough skin-care routine.

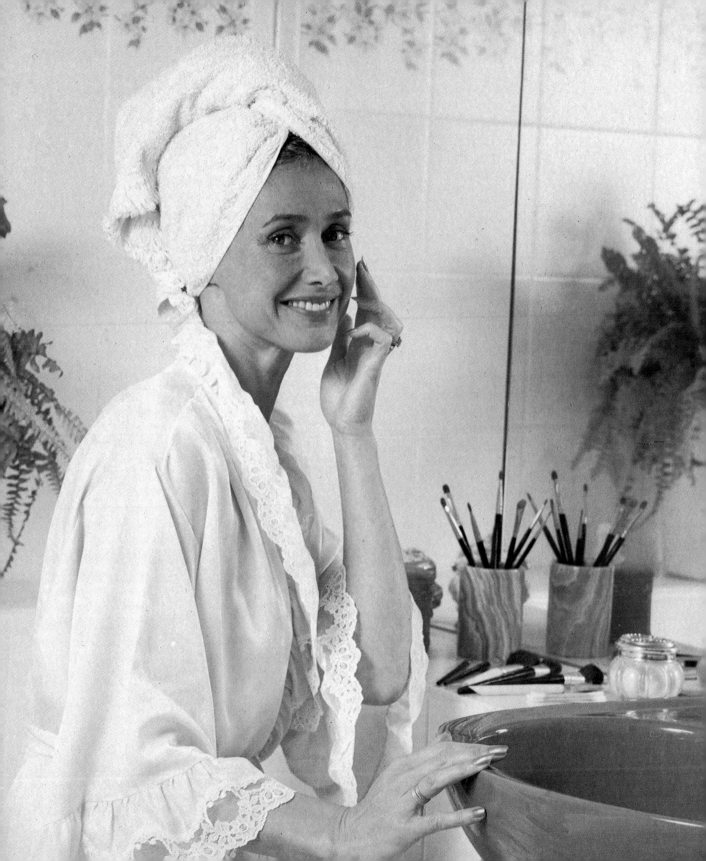

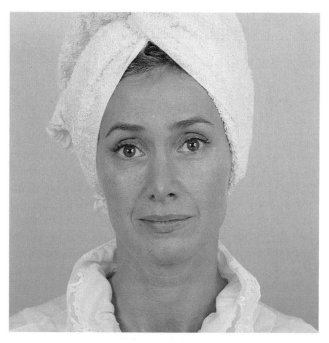

1 After cleansing, toning and moisturizing, my naked face is ready to take make-up.

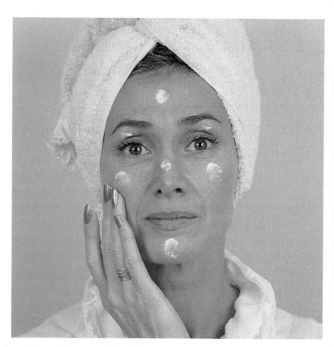

2 I dot a light, liquid foundation on chin, cheeks, nose, forehead and eyelids. Moisturizer has been used here so that you can see it clearly.

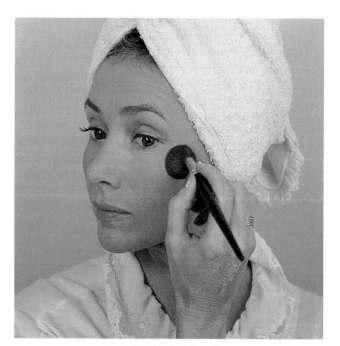

5 After a light dusting of loose face powder – any excess removed with a brush – I apply powder blusher in a warm coral tone. I blend it away from my cheeks and upward towards the temples.

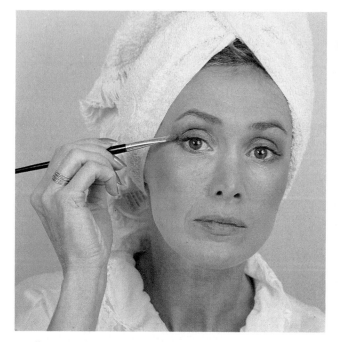

6 All eye products should be first applied to the hand to remove excess and avoid smudging on the eyes. I emphasize my eyes by enhancing the crease with a brown powder shadow and using a thin line of black eyeliner close to the top lashes.

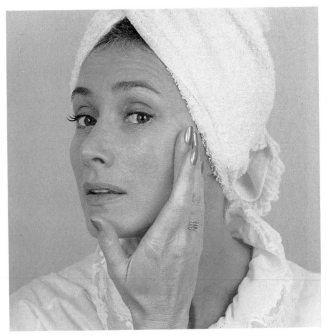

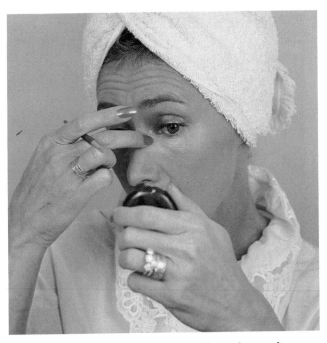

3 My foundation tone is warm but close to my own skin tone. Smooth it on with gentle, upward strokes.

4 The dark shadows under my eyes are hidden with concealing cream – applied with a brush and then well blended with the fingers.

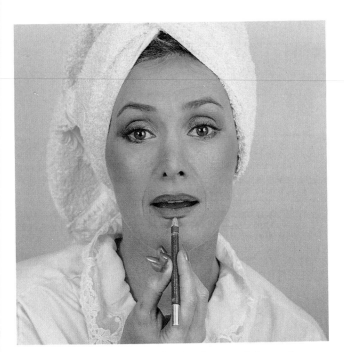

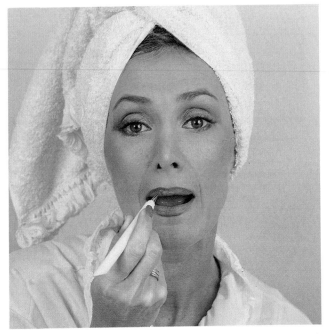

7 Blue powder shadow covers the lid and is extended away from the corners of the my eyes and slightly below. As you can see in the next picture, I sometimes paint a blue line on the lower rim of my eyes before applying mascara.

8 The blue eye-rim line and an outline on the lips with lip pencil can both look rather theatrical for daily use. I apply a warm tone, not a dark colour, of lipstick with a lip brush before a final layer of waterproof mascara (overleaf).

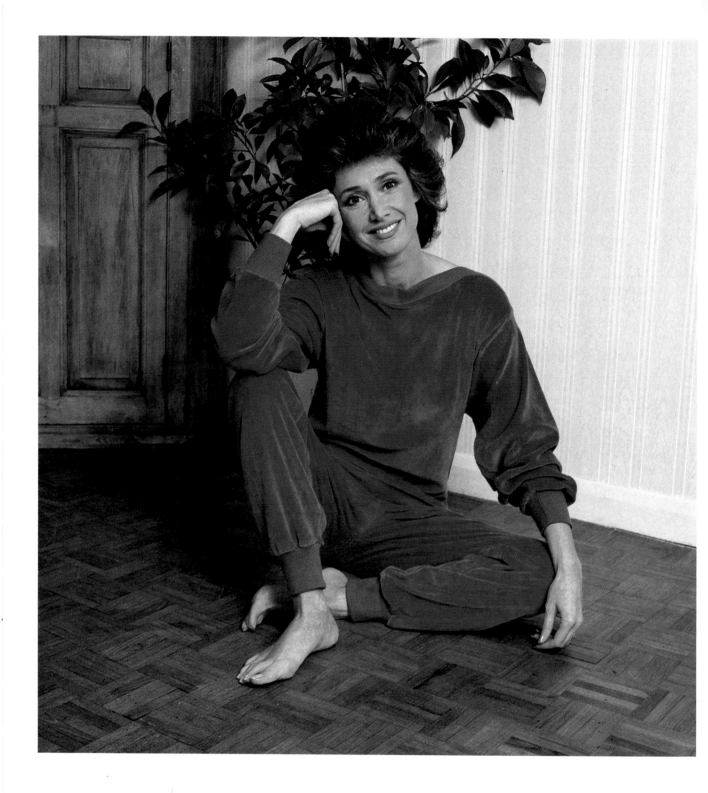

– they dissolve in the blood and tissue fluids and can't be stored in the body for long. Excess is excreted in the urine. Vitamins A, D, E and K are fat soluble. They can be stored for weeks, sometimes months, so even on a poor diet you won't run short for a while.

VITAMIN A: Essential for growth, resistance to infection, eye function – and eating sacks of carrots won't make you see in the dark! Found in liver, eggs, dairy produce, apricots and carrots. Vitamin A is soluble in fat and can be stored in the liver so you don't have to take it every day – most of you are probably taking milk every day anyway, by the glass or in tea and coffee. If you can face liver – many people simply can't – do try and eat some once a week. And don't go mad on the carrots. Apart from not giving you owl vision, an overdose of Vitamin A can be toxic. You could even turn orange!

VITAMIN B$_1$ (THIAMIN): Essential for carbohydrate metabolism. Found in wholemeal bread, lean meat, yeast and wheatgerm. Vitamin B$_1$ can't be stored so you need to ingest it daily. The easiest way is by having a couple of slices of wholemeal toast at breakfast. Incidentally, toast is a few calories less than untoasted bread.

VITAMIN B$_2$ (RIBOFLAVIN): Essential for good skin, nails and hair. Found in milk, cheese, meat, liver, kidneys, yeast and wheatgerm. Vitamin B$_2$ is likely to be found in sufficient quantities in most diets which include dairy products, although it can be destroyed by cooking and light. My milkman calls at such varying hours that I must lose a great deal of the B$_2$ content from my milk – sunshine destroys ten per cent of the riboflavin content hourly. Mind you we don't get that much sunshine!

NICOTINIC ACID: Essential for healthy skin, mucous membranes and the nervous system. Found in bread, liver, meat, fish yeast and wheatgerm. It's less affected by heat and light than other B vitamins but there are losses in overcooking.

VITAMIN B$_6$: Essential for good skin and proper growth in children. Found in liver and kidneys. And if you simply can't stand offal or you're vegetarian, take it in tablet form. Incidentally, it has been suggested that the contraceptive pill leads to a depletion in vitamin B$_6$ – so a supplement is a good idea.

PANTOTHENIC ACID: Essential for helping to burn fat and for fluid balance. Found in liver, beans and yeast.

FOLIC ACID AND VITAMIN B$_{12}$ (CYANOCOBALAMIN): Essential for healthy blood. Folic acid is found in liver, milk, green vegetables and yeast. Vitamin B$_{12}$ is found in liver and meat.

VITAMIN C (ASCORBIC ACID): Essential for resistance to disease, healthy bones, teeth, blood vessels and vitality. Found in green vegetables, potatoes and citrus fruit. It can't be stored in the body and losses during cooking are enormous – up to seventy per cent for green vegetables. Yet another case for only par-cooking your vegetables if you must cook them. Better still, eat them raw.

VITAMIN D (CHOLECALCIFEROL): Essential for regulating the phosphorus and calcium content of the body and bone formation in children. Not that long ago in this country, one could see the sad results of Vitamin D deficiency in the deformed legs of people who'd had rickets as children. Found in fishliver oils, eggs, milk and sunshine. It can be stored in the liver so a weekly helping of the aforementioned is fine provided you get some sun too. In the winter, a cod liver oil capsule daily is a good idea.

VITAMIN E (TOCOPHEROL): Essential for protection of body tissue and blood circulation. Found in wholewheat bread, nuts, vegetable oils and wheatgerm. It can also be used in oil form externally to treat dry skin and wrinkles.

VITAMIN K: Essential to produce blood-clotting. Found in tomatoes, soya bean oil, carrot tops, dark green leafy vegetables and the ubiquitous liver.

I've given you this list of vitamins, not only so that you should know better what your body requires, but also so that if you think you're short on any of them, you can take a vitamin supplement. See how often liver crops up and yet it is certainly not a dish to everyone's taste.

Minerals

The importance of minerals in our body metabolism is a fairly recent discovery. They work by triggering off the action of vitamins in our body. There are about twenty minerals in our body.

IRON: Found in red meat, egg yolks, and good old liver again.

CALCIUM: Found in milk, cheese and yoghurt – vital for bone formation even in adult life. Especially necessary for children as their bones are forming and for pregnant women, where the baby drains the mother of her own calcium.

Other essential minerals are magnesium and phosphorus, sodium, potassium, chloride, iodine and zinc. To ensure that we take in all these essential minerals, it is important that we eat a wide variety of foods.

Good food – how to eat it

Working out the ingredients for a balanced diet is none too difficult but adjusting your eating patterns is. If you have a number of mouths to feed – and mouths which demand sweet, starchy instant food – a limited budget and little time for planning menues, shopping and cooking, then life can become very difficult. Almost everyone who enjoys cooking likes to undertake special meals, dinner parties and party food. However, having to provide three meals a day for the family is a far more demanding and less rewarding task. Making sure there is variety as well as good nutritional value can be difficult. Convenience food is important to many women because they do not have the time or the energy to create wholefood masterpieces every day. I have already said that white bread should be avoided but a house full of growing adolescents screaming for food and wanting endless snacks of cheese on toast or bread, butter and marmite can take the charm out of cutting slices of wholemeal bread. (Most bakeries do now slice large wholemeal loaves, which helps).

However, the key is balance and there are various ways of ensuring you and your family eat well without spending your entire time in the kitchen. Fill them up on potatoes cooked in their skins, on brown rice, wholemeal pasta and so on, so that they do not demand stodgy puddings – give them a delicious fruit yoghurt instead or try and wean them on to fresh fruit. Try and serve at least one fresh vegetable every day – maybe supplemented with a frozen one. But do not overcook them. Better still, serve a salad each day – not so easy in winter.

Cut down on the amount of salt you use in cooking – again it takes time but taste buds do alter to enjoy the real taste of the food rather than the salt.

Sugar is another enemy to be cut down as much as possible – be it brown, white or rainbow colours. Many 'savoury' foods have added sugar – frozen peas for example. That's why children love them so. Soft drinks are usually very high in sugar. Try and buy drinks without additives, they are becoming more readily available. Try using honey as an alternative sweetener in cooking and drinks – it is far better for you than refined sugar.

Do not overcook vegetables – if you do you might as well not bother cooking them. The vitamin content will drop dramatically. The very best way to cook vegetables is to steam them – it is rather more time-consuming but they remain crunchy and delicious.

Having tried just about everything in the book for the broken veins in my feet, I finally visited a homeopathic doctor. I was pleased that he approved of my overall food regime and interested when he said that nowadays a great many of trace elements and minerals are disappearing from our food because of the way it is produced. However good our diet, most of us need a few extra vitamins and minerals – me in particular. I'm now swallowing them as though they are going out of fashion. I can't report any major improvement in my feet (the vitamins are supposed to get my sluggish system working better so that the blood pushed down into the feet, does what it should and comes back up again instead of lying around disfiguring me) but I haven't had a cold for ages while everyone around me is going down like nine-pins. And, though I've been working exceptionally hard and making do on a minimum of sleep, I feel tremendous. Before you rush out and spend money on extra vitamins, *do consult your doctor.*

The best way to get the minerals and trace elements necessary to a healthy diet is to have a salad every day. I now keep a permanent supply of salad stuff in my fridge varying according to season. It's much more difficult to sit down to a salad in the winter but I keep on telling myself that it's doing me good. In fact, I now eat my salad at lunchtime and avoid the sort of convenience foods I very often succumbed to – cheese and biscuits or beans on toast.

Jan's Salad

STOCK:

> *Iceberg lettuce or white cabbage, shredded*
> *tomatoes*
> *pepper (green or red)*
> *button mushrooms*
> *carrots*

These are the basic ingredients to which can be added anything in the salad line which takes your fancy. If you like them add radishes, beans, cucumber, etc. Nuts and sultanas aren't forbidden unless you are dieting.

DRESSING:

> *Olive oil, two parts*
> *cider vinegar, one part*
> *runny honey to taste – not a potful!*
> *salt and pepper*
> *garlic, if you like it – I do.*

Don't put them all on a plate separated like bashful teenagers at a party – do what the Mediterraneans do – cut everything, except the lettuce which should be broken, into small cubes and mix together in a salad bowl. The juices from the ingredients mix and make for an altogether more interesting salad. Then pour over the dressing. If you're having it as a snack, try some cottage cheese with it.

Do you have a weight problem?

I get irritated by people who say, 'You're alright, you don't have a weight problem. You're so slim.' As I've described, and you can see from some of my earlier photographs, I was once overweight and I have no intention of travelling down that path again.

In some ways people who say those with naturally slim figures are lucky, are correct. The main reason I maintain a slim figure is that I am lucky enough to have seen the light and I altered my eating habits. I have a very active life and I am certain that I now have a faster metabolism than previously.

Body fat accumulates when the food you eat, your source of energy, is greater than the amount of energy you use up. In its normal day-to-day functioning, essential to keep you alive, the body uses large amounts of your food intake. It does this in enabling the body to carry out such basic functions as breathing and circulating the blood. The rate at which your body uses up energy in these functions is your basic metabolic rate. It is estimated that about two thirds of your food intake is used in this way. More is used in physical exertion – be it stretching to yawn or jogging.

What all this comes down to is that if you have a fast metabolic rate then most of the food you eat is taken up before you so much as move a muscle. If you have a slow metabolic rate then excess energy, or food intake, turns to fat if it is not burned off by physical activity. It takes an enormous amount of physical activity to use it up. If you tend to be chubby you can reduce your excess fat by reducing your intake of food, particularly highly calorific food, and by increasing exercise. Hence slimming and exercise are recommended for trimming **a** full figure.

Recent research has shown that people who are regular dieters, particularly crash dieters, but who find that they regain weight quickly when they return to normal eating, may in fact be slowing down their metabolic rate by dieting too often. Dieting can lead to a lack of energy and general sloth. It is fairly obvious, and certainly true for me, that in the long term it is necessary to regulate your food intake to suit your energy requirements. Crash diets will reduce weight in the short term but have no lasting effect. Sticking to a sensible overall eating plan, avoiding highly fattening food if you tend to put on weight, and taking regular exercise, are essential.

I say healthy, not thin. It is not fashionable to be large or to have a good covering of flesh. It is fashionable to be slim. However, slim and thin are not the same thing. It can be just as unhealthy, and unattractive, to be too thin as it is to be overweight. If you are feeling healthy and firm, and you cannot therefore grab handfuls of flesh from your body, then you are almost certainly not overweight. But you may not be the shape, naturally, that you think is fashionable and desirable.

How many times have you confronted a woman who, in your opinion, has a good figure but who declares that she has a weight problem? She is not lying, merely insecure about her body shape. Take my sister and me. For years, when I was younger, I envied her figure. She is shorter than I am, about five feet two inches, and has a very small bottom. She looks great in trousers. She has an ample bust and is generally trim. I have small bones, though I am taller, a small bust and, I think, I look lousy in trousers because I have a shapely bottom. Now I realize that we are both lucky in having good figures; we are simply built differently.

You have to learn to live with your build. Some small-boned women have an ample covering of flesh, some don't. If you are desperately trying to rid yourself of flesh which is part of your natural shape, and in proportion and attractive, then why bother? Others have large frames and little excess fat but still try and lose inches. You cannot lose inches off bones even if you starve yourself!

The size and shape of your body is only one factor in your overall appearance. If you are relaxed and happy about your body, a part of being confident about yourself as a person, then you probably look more attractive than those who are not. If you like your body, whatever shape it is, then you are more likely to clothe it well and look after it, including your complexion and hair. Do accept what you are. If you are naturally small, naturally large or naturally curvaceous, then eat sensibly, dress appropriately and you will appear far more attractive than someone who is basically unhappy about how she looks. Someone who squeezes into clothes a size too small, who lives on nothing but diet cola and slimming biscuits, who cares little about health except for frantic bursts of exercise to lose weight, that someone is her own worse enemy. She is trying to be someone she is not rather than making the best of what she has got.

Weight problems

I am not suggesting that fat is good for you. If you are overweight, even if you like being fat, it is not good for you. If you carry a large amount of excess fat you are putting an extra stress on your heart, lungs, legs, everything. I once said to a doctor friend how very sorry I felt for fat people. 'Don't,' he retorted. 'With the few exceptions of those with glandular problems, really fat people eat too much and don't get enough exercise.' In fact, he was running a scheme to get tonnage off the populace of the village in which he lived. He was doing very well too, with the exception of one fat biddy. Every time she came the scales stayed stubbornly at the same weight. Every week the doctor asked her if she was adhering to the diet sheet. Every week, she said that she most definitely was being a good girl. Finally, in exasperation, as she was leaving the surgery one evening he suggested that she must be nibbling in between meals. 'Oh no, doctor,' she said, her little red cheeks breaking into a smile 'the only extra I have is my pot of honey a day!' Honey is extremely good for you but not by the potful and not when you're overweight!

In my early twenties, I was domiciled in Australia, earning my living as an actress. At one stage I joined a very small touring company to take 'potted' Shakespeare to the outlying districts of New South Wales. We covered 17,000 miles in seven months, performing at least twice a day, except Sundays, and very often travelling hundreds of miles over make-shift roads in between venues. That was when I got fat, not totally my own fault. We were working hard, living on not too much money and very often dependant on the hospitality of the various Arts Councils in the areas we visited. Time and time again, lunch was sandwiches and cakes, instead of the salads we would have eaten had we had the time to go and forage for ourselves, and the money. Often we'd have hours to fill after arriving in a place and before we gave a performance. We couldn't afford comfortable hotels and the places in which we stayed were literally just for sleeping in. So we'd repair to the local coffee bar and drink cups and cups of revolting flavoured milk, which the proprietors called coffee, and dig into more cakes and other fat-inducing foods. To be fair, nearly twenty years ago, it was much more difficult to 'eat well' than it is today.

The tour ended and we got back to Sydney. My agent rang me excitedly and said I was to have a meeting with a producer at the ABC (equivalent to the BBC) for a lead part in a play. The producer, French by birth, entered the room and all he said was 'You 'ave put on weight' – end of interview, collapse of stout party – me. While on tour I had let out the belt on my uniform skirt and I'd noticed that my blouse was rather tight but I hadn't actually got onto the scales. I'd gone from about eight and a half stone to just under ten. Nothing wrong with that except that I'm five feet five inches tall and small-boned. I didn't look gross but I felt as if I was carrying round sacks of coal with me.

Of course, I didn't get the part and was mortified when I found that all the clothes I'd left in Sydney simply didn't fit. Shifts were the only thing that hid the fat.

I embarked on diet after diet, even used slimming pills – which I *do not* recommend. I'd get some weight off, then put some back on again. I was very disheartened. I loathe dieting. I like food, tasty food. I'll eat salads with home-made salad dressing but when lunch was a lettuce leaf, half a tomato and no dressing, I'd be ravenous before dinner. I tried the steak, egg and wine diet and just felt tipsy. I read so many calorie charts that to this day, although I couldn't give you exact numbers, I have an in-built computer which tells me what I can and can't eat.

How did I beat the flab? Finally it was a combination of an emotional upset which got the weight off (I don't recommend this course either) and eating everything I wanted that was not horrendously fattening. I ate only small quantities, never having seconds, cutting out the bread rolls if I was taken to dinner, and never touched dessert unless it was a piece of fresh fruit. I cut down on wine – I've never been a great drinker of spirits anyway – and if I was at a drinks gathering, I'd have tonic water. (Nowadays, I very often have a sparkling mineral water. Everyone thinks you're drinking a gin and tonic and they don't pester you to have a real drink.) I lost a stone in weight. Over the years, with sensible eating and, no doubt, the stresses imposed on me by my work, I got down to the weight I wanted to be, around the eight stone mark, and with the exception of having my son, Jonathan, have remained at a constant weight now for the last fourteen years.

I'm not telling you this because I think I deserve a pat on the back but because I firmly believe that you have to *re-adjust your approach to eating* to lose weight in the long term.

Do I ever indulge in cream cakes and more than one glass of wine? Of course I do. But I play a game of reward and punishment with myself. When I've indulged in a meal, or meals, which I know have more calories than are necessary to sustain me, then I compensate for it on the next day at home when I can eat what I like or don't like. Then I'm strict and eat less calories in a day than I'm allowed. That way, I even the balance. I also weigh myself every day and if, for whatever reason, the arrow has crept up a pound or two, I watch what I eat until those offending pounds have gone. It's the only way to do it – if you wait until your belt is pinching, you've probably put on something like five to seven pounds – that's equivalent to three large bags of sugar. And that amount of weight is a darned sight harder to shift than the odd pound.

Serious weight problems

If you are seriously overweight and you know you need major weight loss, you must consult your doctor. Remember that initially the weight will come off quickly if you're following a healthy diet, but the last stone to half-stone will be very difficult to shift. If you're drastically overweight by stones rather than pounds, then be prepared for at least a year of hard work to get down to a reasonable size. I know I'm painting a black picture but if you go on crash diets and lose weight quickly, a lot of weight I'm talking about, your skin will go flabby, you won't be all that healthy, and what's more important when you come off the 'crash' diet you'll start putting the weight back on again. It took years to put it on, be patient in getting it off. Give yourself goals – I'll be down one size in six months and treat myself to a few new clothes – not too many because, we hope, you'll be discarding them after a season to go to a size smaller and so on. Remember, *everything in moderation*.

If you find dieting a lonely occupation, you can join an organization such as Weight Watchers where you'll have the companionship of other 'biggies' and you'll have regular goals to attain. The Weight Watchers' regime is based on what I'm talking about – good, tasty, interesting food but the *right* food. Your taste buds must be satisfied or you will crave food. When I'm home and can eat what I like, I never nibble. At work, where I have to eat whatever is on offer at the canteen, which rarely satisfies my taste buds, I find myself eating unmentionables by the end of the day – dreadful things like chocolate bars. And don't I know it when the little spots come out a few days later.

If you are aiming to lose a great deal of weight, you should have a regular exercise routine as well to help firm your muscles. Again, check with your doctor before embarking on anything strenuous.

SOME DO'S AND DON'TS FOR SLIMMING

DO consult your doctor if you are aiming at large weight loss. Also consult him about supplementary vitamins and minerals.

DO remember that persistent triers succeed in reaching their goals. If at first you don't succeed try, try and try again. A perfectionist may be disillusioned and fail in the attempt.

DO remember that some foods may be high in calories but rich in vitamins. Avocados are highly calorific but they are packed with Vitamin E and also quite filling. Lunch of half an avocado, a nice big one, with some prawns is most satisfying. If prawns aren't to your taste, use tuna fish, cottage cheese, taramasalata – anything you fancy.

DO drink a lot of water. Mineral water is best because our tap water these days is re-cycled so much. But if you do drink tap water, run it for a time in the morning to get rid of the metallic particles it may have picked up from lying in the pipes. Water is purifying and in large quantities, does take the edge off hunger.

DO weigh yourself regularly – every day is best – then you'll be aware of any unwanted poundage before it becomes too acute.

DO remember that the more active the life you lead, the less you'll be tempted to nibble. Boredom, too much time on your hands, they're the culprits that tempt you to indulge in more food than you need, and the wrong food at that.

DO think HEALTH. If you're slimming, once you reach your target weight, there's very little that you'll have to forego totally. Remember, all the good food you want, in *moderation*. It will take time to re-think your approach to food but I promise you it can and does work. You'll even be able to allow yourself the odd cream cake but I'll take a bet with you that you won't often desire it.

DON'T slim for someone else. The motivation must be yours alone. If you're slimming for your husband, lover or boyfriend, the moment the poor soul overlooks your efforts, you're likely to say 'What's the use' and slip back into your bad old ways.

DON'T forget the difference between self-control and will-power. If your will-power slips and you eat a chocolate bar, you'll probably feel you've blown it and give up the whole idea. With self-control you'll know that there will be the odd lapses but they are not terminal, and the occasional fall from grace is not going to ruin your whole diet.

DON'T see a 'binge' as anything other than a momentary lapse – this applies when you get to your target weight too. If you've had a binge, *compensate* the next day or two.

DON'T put temptation in your way unnecessarily. By that I mean – avoid your favourite cake shop – don't go and look in the window and drool. Don't keep at home the foods you know are bad for you but which you find hard to resist. I never keep cake in the house.

Essential check-ups

Years ago, when I first began reporting and interviewing for television, I was sent out to do a Vox Pop – a street interview where a stranger approaches you, shoves a microphone at you and asks a question. The subject was the relatively new Cervical Smear Test. Many of the women interviewed didn't know what it was and I patiently explained it to them pointing out that if the worst happened and cervical cancer was detected early, treatment was virtually one hundred per cent effective. I was horrified at the percentage of women who said they wouldn't want to know.

Every woman should have a regular Cervical Smear Test. The first test is followed by another after a year and then at three-year intervals. There's nothing to it. The doctor inserts a small plastic instrument called a speculum into the vagina. He takes a smear from the cervix which is placed on a slide. This goes to a cytologist who analyzes it under a microscope. The results are back within one to six weeks according to the workload at the laboratory. Detected and treated early, there is a very high cure rate for cancer of the cervix.

You should also examine your breasts regularly, the best time being immediately after a period. If you test just before, very often you find little lumps and bumps which are nothing whatever to do with cancer, just the body reacting to hormone changes. If you're past the age of periods just do an examination on a regular day each month.

Obviously your doctor will give you a breast examination but you shouldn't really expect him or her to do it monthly. They'll show you how to do it, if you're having difficulty.

Here are the six steps to self-examination. If you have anything that worries you, go immediately to your doctor. You'll probably find that it's a non-malignant cyst but if it's anything worse, early detection is essential and early treatment gives the best chance of cure.

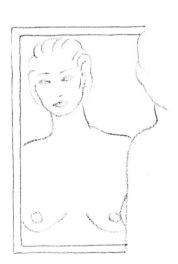

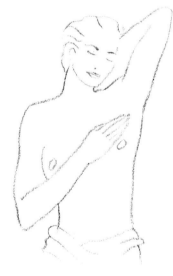

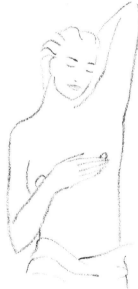

Breast self-examination
First study your breasts in the mirror for any change in size or appearance, any puckering or dimpling in the skin. Then raise your arms above your head, and turn from side to side, studying the sides of your breasts for any changes. Check the nipples for any bleeding or unusual discharge.

Lie down and put your left hand behind your head. Think of your breast as being divided into four quarters of a circle, and start the examination with the upper inner quarter. Using the flat of the fingers of the right hand, work from well out from the breast towards the nipple, feeling for anything unusual.

Working inwards on the lower inner quarter.

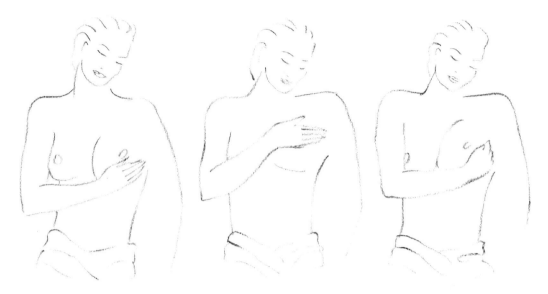

Bring your left arm down to your side and examine the lower outer quarter.

Working inwards on the upper outer quarter.

Finally feel in the armpit for any lumps. And now repeat the whole examination on the other breast.

Smoking

Do try to give it up. It's a dirty, anti-social habit, and even worse it does untold damage to your skin. There is a substance called benzopyrene found in cigarette smoke which uses up the body's vital supply of Vitamin C. Vitamin C supports the collagen in your skin and without it the skin wrinkles early. Here's a horrendous fact – the skin of smokers wrinkles and ages up to twenty years sooner than that of non-smokers. Unfortunately, non-smokers cannot escape the deleterious effects of other people's smoking – all the more reason to try and persuade your friends and loved ones not to smoke in your house. In a room of smokers the carbon monoxide level from the leftover cigarette smoke can be as much as twenty to eighty parts per million. In industry the acceptable level of this poisonous gas is fifty parts per million! Carbon monoxide inhibits the red blood cells oxygen carrying capacity leading to oxygen starvation. Without this all important substance, your body can't break down the nutrients to produce energy and in turn nourish the cells. Smoking is also a contributory factor to heart disease, strokes and bronchial ailments. DO GIVE IT UP.

If you simply can't then take Vitamin C supplementary to your diet but this won't *stop* the premature ageing of the skin, it will only help a little.

Sleep

We all need sleep in varying amounts. Some people can get by quite happily on four or five hours sleep a night, older folk need less sleep and some like me are eight hour people. This has become very difficult to achieve with a small child who wakes at an earlier time than I am used to getting up. Before my son was born, I would go to bed late, usually around 1 am and rise late. Now, if I want to get more than six hours I have to start heading for bed at what to me seems to be the early hour of 10 pm.

Whatever your sleep requirement is, do try and achieve it. If you've had a lot of late nights, pamper yourself by going to bed really early and catching up on your sleep. And if you do have a sleepless night every now and then, don't worry about it. We all go through periods when our minds simply won't switch off and the more we toss and turn the less likely we are to fall asleep. If you're having a bad night, try doing the stretching and relaxing pregnancy exercises described in the next chapter, they may not send you to sleep but they should calm you so that you can at least benefit by being in bed and having a rest.

To help you sleep

1 Do have a window open if at all possible; stuffy air does nothing to help you sleep.
2 Do take a milk drink if you feel a bit edgy and think you might not sleep. Milk is high in calcium and induces muscle relaxation.
3 If you can't drink milk, how about herb tea with a spoonful of honey. The best teas for sleep inducement are camomile, skullcap, peppermint and vervain. They take a little getting used to but with anything like that I tell myself it's doing me good and soldier on until I eventually develop a taste for it.
4 If you bathe at night, take your bath immediately before bed. Make sure it's lukewarm. A hot bath will stimulate your heart and be no help at all.
5 Don't drink alcohol too close to bedtime. If you're out at a function, have a glass of wine with the meal and then go onto mineral water. Drink does put you to sleep but you'll always wake in the small hours, dehydrated, feeling awful and totally unable to go back to sleep again. If you do have several drinks at dinner, then make sure you drink at least a pint of water when you get home.
6 Don't drink coffee late at night. I do have a few friends who can drink coffee

immediately prior to bed and still sleep but most of us can't. If you've got to have a coffee after your dinner, drink the decaffeinated variety.

7 Don't go to bed when you're not sleepy just because you feel you ought to. Read a book. If circumstances and weather allow it, take a walk before bed.

When you're sleeping your internal organs have a chance to rest. Most tension, unless it's really deep-seated, will disappear overnight. Your body cells are revitalized and you will find that after a good night's sleep your eyes have more sparkle and your skin looks better. Sleep is the least expensive beauty aid you can get.

Teeth

You should visit your dentist every six months for a check-up and a clean. The plaque that builds up around your teeth near the gums is not only unsightly and smelly, but it's hiding a whole lot of trouble that could be building up in your gums. As we get older our gums recede fast enough without allowing the plaque to have a field day! Where plaque builds up, the gums are soft and where they are soft, they recede even more quickly. You should brush your teeth twice, if not three times a day, properly – not just a quick swish around the mouth. If you can't be bothered to clean for about two minutes, then treat yourself to an electric toothbrush and let that take the elbow-grease out of cleaning. You should then use dental floss in between your teeth, at least once a day. This is something that your dentist should show you. It isn't difficult but it's very easy to pull the wrong way and get the floss stuck. And for goodness sake, change your toothbrush at least once a month – they were not designed to last a lifetime!

My two front teeth used to go inwards like rabbit teeth and they had a strange mark on them caused by some illness as an infant, and next to them was a half-tooth – I'd let it go so far that it was nearly all filling. They were a source of embarassment to me and it wasn't until my mid-twenties that I had anything done about them. I have three crowns in the front of my mouth and I only wish I'd had them done years before when I was a gawky, self-conscious teenager.

False teeth

If you have them do get them checked every few years. One set doesn't last a lifetime, or shouldn't do. Your jaw changes shape as you age and the gums recede. If you're still clinging onto the set you first had it's highly likely you are getting those little age lines around your mouth where the lips have nothing to plump them up (like the collagen in your skin). This was beginning to happen to a friend of mine. Off she went to the dentist, got a new set of teeth which helped to plump out the lips, and the lines have disappeared.

Dental correction

If your teeth are crooked, jumbled together, seriously stained or chipped, to the extent that it distresses you, then have a word with your dentist. You might find that it is an extreme enough case to be treated under the National Health. Failing that, if you do have to pay yourself, isn't it worth going without a few items of clothes for one season in order to have a pretty mouth?

Health hydros

In the interests of writing this book, and purely out of a sense of duty, you understand, I felt that I had to experience a health hydro. Being a consumate believer in the 'small is beautiful' theory, I headed down to my beloved West Country and to a newly-opened establishment with twenty-nine rooms catering for around forty guests.

I went with an open mind and a full suitcase. The suitcase was unnecessary – everyone drifted around in towelling robes, tracksuits, leotards and no one dressed for dinner.

The old idea of a health farm was predominately a place where one went in order to shed pounds. Although they will help you to do this in a hydro, it would be more accurate to describe it as an establishment for a body service – just like a car service. Although there were some overweight people around, there were others with very good bodies who had just come to have a de-coke – there were one or two good-looking couples too. Are men such male chauvinist pigs that they don't think we mind about their spreading middles and pot bellies – why is it always the women who are trying to improve themselves. Needless to say, there were hardly any men in attendance.

I had gone for a bit of rest and relaxation, didn't need to lose weight and could have eaten normal meals. However, as I didn't have the pressure of work, I decided to go on a de-toxification diet for twenty-four hours to try and get the toxins out of my system. This consisted of half a pineapple and fresh orange juice for breakfast, lunch and dinner with the odd glass of juice, if I wanted it, mid-morning and mid-afternoon. It was surprisingly satisfying.

Those who came to lose weight, had a consultation with the principal – a trained

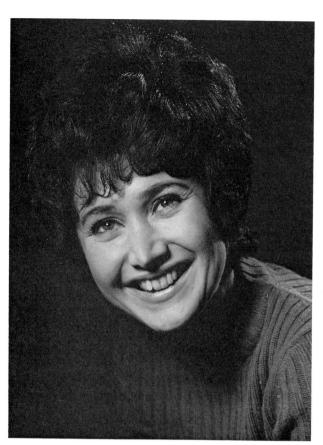

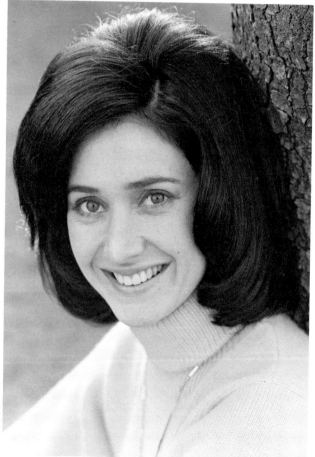

nurse who had also done courses and worked with homeopathy, osteopathy, and naturapathy. She assesses your condition and decides whether you can tolerate a fast for a day or even two. If you don't need to lose weight, you can still have a consultation and decide what sort of food you're going to eat. After my de-toxification day, I went onto salads – and delicious they were too. There are four-day stays and seven-day stays and prices range from £173 per person for seven days on a budget rate, through Standard, Premier and Executive rooms to Suites at £65 per person per day, roughly the price of a room in an hotel. But whether you're staying in the best or the least expensive room, *every* guest has four treatments a day which are included in the price – the treatments being a manual massage, a G5 massage (with machine), a Faradic massage (machine for muscle toning) and a sauna or a steam bath. There's unlimited use of the swimming pool, jacuzzi, and gymnasium, and guests can also take advantage of keep fit and movement to music classes. There are also other extras for which one pays – facials, manicures, pedicures, hairdressing, peat baths and mud packs.

For those who haven't the time or can't afford four days or a week, the hydro offers 'Top to Toe' days for four treatments and use of the pool and jacuzzi.

During my stay, a party of women came for a 'Top to Toe' and extra staff had to be enlisted to cater for the massages etc. One recruit was a young man – most of the massage is usually done by females. A group of us were waiting and the lady next to me was allocated to the male masseur. She didn't look too happy about it! I offered to swap and received the best massage I've ever had in my life. I suffer from tension in my shoulders, a state of health which often leads to very severe headaches. This young man felt my muscle tension immediately and really went to work with a vengeance on my shoulders. The relief was superb – I felt so relaxed I could have fallen asleep there and then but it was lunchtime and I was really looking forward to my salad.

Most health farms and hydros are established in old country houses with spacious grounds, mine was no exception. It was a lovely and gracious building with a great deal of oak panelling, a feeling of space and lovely grounds in which to walk, sit, or even play nine holes of golf. I went with an open mind and left after two and a half days feeling fitter, very relaxed and a total convert. I had also lost three pounds in weight. A few days at a hydro, a health holiday, will now feature prominently in my plans when I'm arranging my diary for the year.

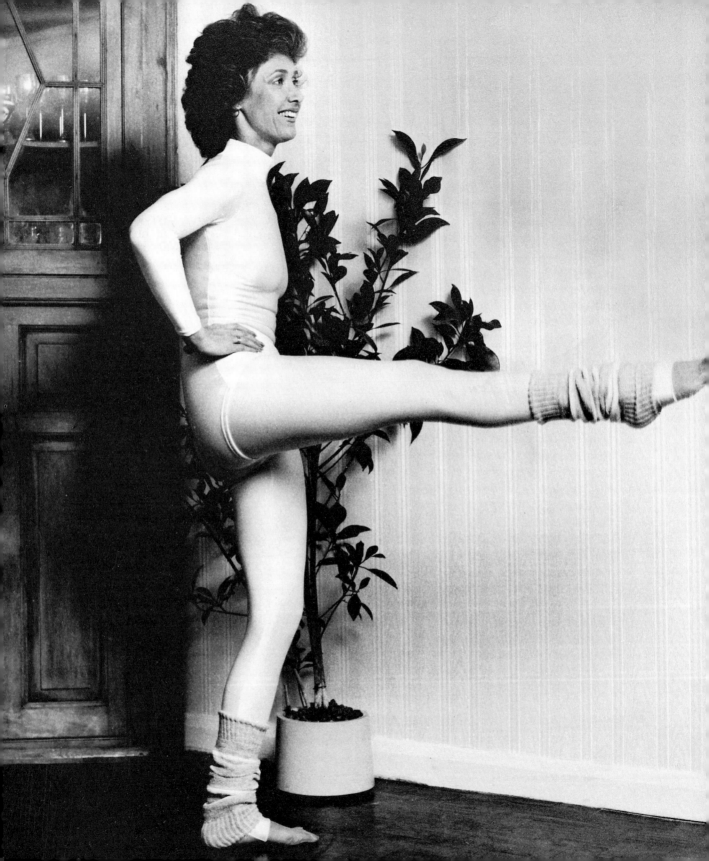

Exercise

I must confess that I find exercise a rather boring occupation. By that I mean exercise routines, done alone at home. However, I breathed a sigh of relief when exercise to music tapes appeared. I love dancing and music and what could be better than swapping dance steps for an exercise routine. I had been rather daunted by the advent of aerobics and very strenuous routines. I lead an extremely active life, and a busy one, so the thought of putting aside long periods of time in order to thoroughly exhaust myself has never seemed particularly attractive.

However, exercise is extremely important and while I cannot claim to be an enthusiast I would encourage anyone to have a go and find something they enjoy doing without unduly straining the body. Do not be put off exercise altogether because you think you have to jump straight in at the deep end and thrash your body into shape and health.

One of the easiest ways to exercise is to indulge in some sport like tennis or squash. Unfortunately I am hopeless at most sports. I tried so hard at school but it was as if I met a gremlin at every sports period – suffering black and blue legs from hockey, a knock on the head from a rounders bat and a tennis ball in the eye which broke a blood vessel. I was thrown from a horse when I tried to learn to ride a few years ago, almost split myself in two trying to waterski and made a mess of snow skiing. It's not that I haven't tried!

The one sporty activity I love is swimming and it is in fact perhaps the best activity for exercising because it affects every single muscle in your body. I am none too brilliant a swimmer either but I can manage a few lengths and I thoroughly enjoy it. That is the key to exercise, find something you enjoy, that you can do easily and that makes you feel good.

Why exercise

It strengthens the heart – the most important muscle in your body. If you've ever suffered a broken limb you will know how quickly muscle wastes.

It increases circulation – which in turn increases the nourishment to the body.

It makes joints more flexible, and you more supple.

It firms flesh in the right places.

It makes you feel better. The increased blood circulation plus your oxygen intake (the lungs are working harder, expanding and taking in more oxygen) all contribute to a feeling of well-being.

In firming your body, you will lose a few inches, but it is not to be seen as a weight reducer.

If your body is more supple, you will hold yourself better and improve your posture. Good posture in itself aids breathing, and puts less strain on the spine.

It keeps your blood–sugar levels from fluctuating dramatically. When muscles are exercised regularly they oxidize an increased amount of fat from the body, using less of your body's carbohydrate (sugar and starch). It is when your blood–sugar level drops that you feel hunger.

It increases movement in the intestines. The time for food to travel through your body and be excreted is diminished – therefore your body absorbs fewer calories.

In brief, exercise increases your metabolic rate so that your cells burn oxygen more rapidly and use the nutrients in your food more efficiently, and it improves the removal of waste products from the body. It also makes you less *irritable*. How? We all experience emotional and physical stress which produces adrenalin. If this adrenalin is not used up by exercising, it is stored in your heart and brain affecting your moods and emotion, in turn making you tired and irritable. Even a long walk, when you're feeling uptight, will do you the world of good.

Introducing exercise

Start exercising, if you have not so far indulged, by doing some basic warm-ups and routines at home, or simply as you go through the day. Remember, it's never too late to start but I suggest you start with something simple. The array of exercise routines is mind-boggling so I have asked an expert to set out a simple and basic one for beginners. Alternatively try the bath exercises I suggest, or begin visiting your local swimming pool, do a few lengths and the swimming pool exercises I describe. When you have mastered one, or all, of these you can move on to something more elaborate such as an exercise tape, or join a class.

Bath exercises

A great many people have a little 'soak' in the bath. Instead why not do a few exercises in your 'soaking' time. I suggest you buy one of those rubber mats for the bottom of the bath or you'll probably slip all over the place. A bath pillow is a good idea too. Do the exercises on an empty stomach. Don't have the bathwater too hot – you should never have a too-hot bath under any circumstances. Draw the water to about the half-way mark so that it's up to your neck when you lie back.

TUMMY TIGHTENER: Lie back, knees bent, feet on bottom of the bath, and hands by your sides. Pull in tummy muscles as if you were trying to make your navel touch your spine. Hold for a count of three, then release. It is important to breathe out deeply before you pull in, and breathe in as you release your muscles. Repeat five times.

STRETCH AND STRENGTHEN: This tightens tummy as well as strengthening shoulders, arms, back, hips and legs. (This can only be done if your bath is the right length for you – most modern baths will be but the gorgeous old-fashioned ones will be too roomy). Lie back, legs outstretched and toes wedged under the taps, hands by your sides. Sit up slowly, stretch your arms and try to touch your toes.

If you're not used to exercise, this one will take some time to do properly. Hold for a count of ten, then lie back. You might find you can only do this twice – don't worry – work on it till you can manage to repeat ten times.

THIGH TIGHTENER: Lie back, hands on bottom of bath. Bring right heel towards your bottom. Straighten the leg out again while at the same time bringing your left heel to your posterior. This is more difficult than it sounds. Ideally it should be done ten times with each leg and then ten times with the legs together. But, moderation in all things – if you can only manage it twice, then settle for that for a day or two. If you're unused to exercise, it might take you weeks to achieve the magic ten. Don't worry, don't push yourself too much – *enjoy it*.

WAISTLINE TRIMMER: Sit up, legs slightly apart, feet on bottom of bath. Clasp hands behind head. Twist slowly to the right, as far as is possible. Hold for a count of three, return to original position and relax for three. Now repeat twisting to the left. Repeat whole movement – right and left counts as one movement (no cheating). You should be able to do this ten times.

While on the subject of exercises in water, look at the following ones you can do in the swimming pool to shape up for your summer holiday. You don't have to be a swimmer to do these and the buoyancy of the water makes them easier.

Figure trimming
Although exercise won't lose you very much weight in pounds it will lose you inches as it tones your muscles, keeps you mobile and improves your circulation thereby

Swimming pool exercises
Here are some really effective toning exercises, and of course swimming itself is marvellous. Breast stroke shapes limbs and firms pectoral muscles; back crawl helps shoulders, bust and thighs; front crawl shapes limbs and firms buttocks. Do make sure, after your swim, that you rinse off chemicals or salt under the shower as both are very drying.

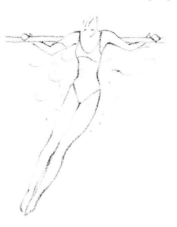

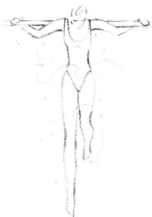

Waist
Holding the bar at the side of the pool, straighten your legs and point your toes. Keep your hands and arms still and gently swing your hips and legs from side to side. The movement should come from the waist, and the legs should remain rigid. Do this for two minutes.

Thighs
With your back to the bar, spread your arms and grip it firmly. Let your body float upwards to just below the surface. Keep the legs straight as you do small scissor movements, never allowing them to break the surface of the water. Do this for two minutes.

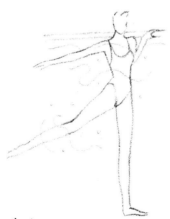

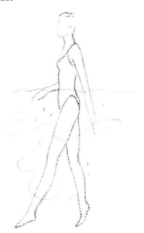

Leg strengthening
Stand in shoulder-high water. Hold the bar with one hand and extend the other arm towards the centre of the pool. Swing the outside leg up as high as you can in front, and then swing it to the back. Repeat four times, then turn and do the other leg.

Stomach flattening
Hold your tummy tight in and walk the width of the shallow end, in waist-high water. Turn round and come back. Speed is impossible but the faster you go the more effective this is.

nourishing the body. I came across two 'movements' which took weight off, quite by accident. Accident was the operative word. I had a contretemps at an accident blackspot with a telegraph pole. My right ankle was smashed and the bone between knee and ankle also suffered. I was in plaster from the knee down with orders not to put any weight on my foot. I lived in a small house in Bristol and of course the loo was upstairs! Many times a day I had to go up and come downstairs on my posterior – at the end of six weeks I had the slimmest hips you could imagine. As the behind and thighs are the places that most women want to lose weight first, why not try going up and downstairs in this slightly ungainly fashion? It's very similar to the hip-banging exercise, you know the one – stand in the corner of the room and bang your hips first on one wall then the other.

The other 'hip slimmer' I discovered was when my son Jonathan was getting mobile at about ten months. Our house was on three storeys with the nursery on the middle floor – that meant two staircases to guard and one of them, being on a bend, did not lend itself to a kiddygate so we put the gate across the nursery door. I don't know how many times a day I had to lift my leg over it, rather than go to the bother of undoing it each time. I still had a few pounds on the hips left over from the pregnancy – they went. I wouldn't suggest putting a kiddygate across the door to the kitchen because you're carrying things, but if you have a room you are constantly going in and out of, then try the gate treatment – lead with your right leg going in and your left leg coming out.

Another amusing way to lose weight, providing your heart is in good condition is by running up and down stairs. A friend of mine told me how, many years ago, when she was doing a bit of local part-time modelling, the show she was engaged for was cancelled, and she went on a bit of an eating binge. I don't know what she ate but she put on about 5 lbs in weight in a week. Then, horrors, she was phoned to say the show was back on again. How was she to lose the weight in double quick time. She ran up and down the stairs over and over again, with a few pauses no doubt. She eventually reached the magic count of sixty and discovered she'd lost the weight she needed to. Rather drastic – but if you're fit, it could be fun.

Breathing

It is essential that you should breathe properly – too many people breathe in a shallow manner which certainly keeps them alive but doesn't get everything moving and circulating inside them.

When you inhale you are taking in a mixture of gases including oxygen which is vital for supplying your body cells. When you exhale you are removing carbon dioxide waste from your system. Well, that's how it should work but many of us do not breathe properly so that the body is neither getting as much oxygen as it needs nor expelling the wastes it should. A percentage of the oxygen you inhale is used directly by your skin and when your skin cells aren't getting the proper supply, they can't carry out their function effectively – cell division slows down and wastes are not removed as they should be. Less than the correct amount of oxygen in your body also affects the functioning of your brain and nerve cells.

Obviously we can't go around deep breathing all day but take a couple of minutes to do it morning and night at least.

Deep breathing involves chest and abdomen. Lie down on a flat surface – your bed or the floor. Put your hands lightly on your stomach and now breathe in. If your hands aren't pushed up by the inhalation of breath, you are not breathing deeply enough. Make a conscious effort to breathe deeply – it will soon come.

Breathe in to a count of five, hold for a count of five, and gradually exhale to a count of five.

Once you know how to breathe properly, it's an idea to do it by an open window – unless you live in the heart of a city in which case you just deep breathe in your room!

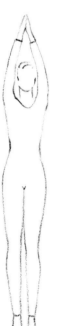

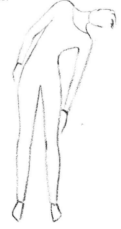

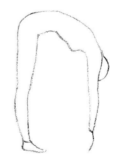

Basic fitness exercise routine
Feet together and arms at sides.
Raise arms to touch fingers high
above head. Repeat ten times.

Feet apart and arms loose at sides,
bend from waist first to one side,
then the other, taking the head
sideways. Repeat ten times.

Feet together and arms at sides.
Flop forward from the waist,
keeping legs straight. Repeat five
times.

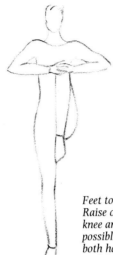

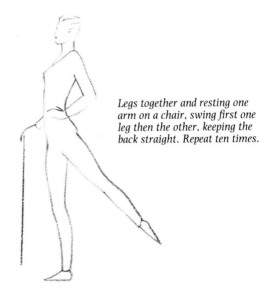

Legs together and resting one arm on a chair, swing first one leg then the other, keeping the back straight. Repeat ten times.

Feet together and arms at sides. Raise one leg, bending at the knee and lifting it as high as possible. Pull the knee in with both hands. Repeat ten times with both legs.

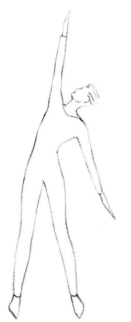

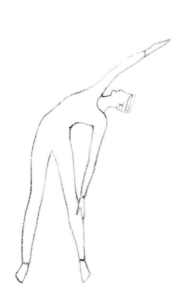

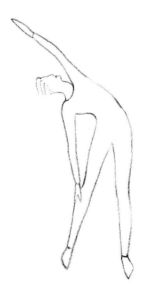

Feet apart and arms at sides. Raise your right arm high, bending body to the left.

Follow through to touch your left knee with your left hand. Hold for a count of five.

Do the last two movements in the opposite direction. Going straight on from one side to the other, repeat the whole exercise five times.

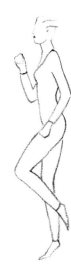

Run on the spot, raising feet as high as possible. Build up to fifty runs.

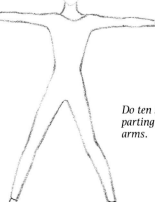

Do ten stride jumps, parting feet and raising arms.

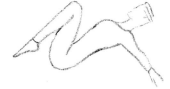

Lie on your back, stretch arms wide from shoulders and raise knees to chest.

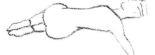

Keeping back and shoulders on the ground, swing knees over to one side.

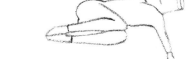

Swing back over the chest to the other side. Repeat whole movement ten times.

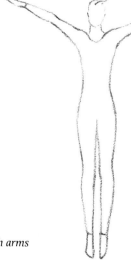

Spring up to a jump, stretching arms. Repeat these two movements ten times, watching your balance when you come down to the crouch.

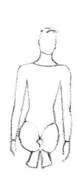

Crouch down with arms at sides.

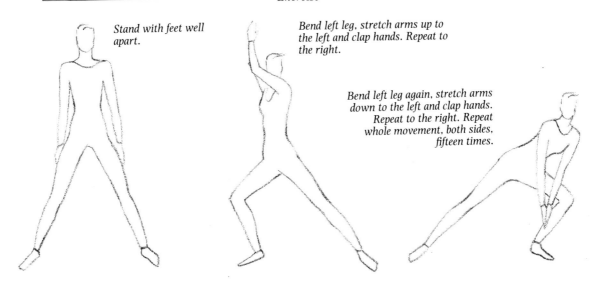

Stand with feet well apart.

Bend left leg, stretch arms up to the left and clap hands. Repeat to the right.

Bend left leg again, stretch arms down to the left and clap hands. Repeat to the right. Repeat whole movement, both sides, fifteen times.

Facial exercises

The face is very often left out of an exercise routine, yet it is the first place to show ageing and requires toning and firming. Many people, and I'm one of them, have deep lines from each corner of the nose to the ends of the mouth. This exercise should stop them getting any worse.

Inhale – close your mouth lightly so that your lips are together but not your teeth. Puff out your cheeks like a frog and hold for a count of five. Open lips slightly and gently blow out all the air. Repeat this exercise fourteen times, once a day. You can do it anywhere – do it whilst you sit and watch television, or at the sink when you're peeling vegetables or washing up.

FOREHEAD: This exercise helps eradicate forehead lines, sagging of the upper eyelid and the small lines at the corner of the eyes. It's not an easy exercise to do but once mastered can be done virtually anywhere.

You have to raise your eyebrows without frowning. Your frontal muscle is raised and when you've mastered the exercise (it may take weeks) there should be no change in the expression on your face. To begin with you'll look startled. Do persevere with this one. It should eventually be done thirty times a day. It can be done anywhere.

CHIN AND THROAT: To tighten chin and throat muscles and keep at bay the double chin; sit at a table, resting your elbows on the edge, close together. Make a fist with each hand and rest chin on fists. Press down with your head and upwards with your fists, continuing the action for about fourteen seconds. Repeat the exercise fourteen times once a day.

Pregnancy and exercise

It is important to exercise during pregnancy and particularly if you are an older mother-to-be. I had my first baby at thirty-nine and there wasn't one single bit of me that seemed elderly. I felt superbly well, apart from the few weeks of morning sickness which were soon controlled with medication, and immensely happy. Every mother owes it to herself to do relaxation exercises in the run-up period to labour and birth. If she is relaxed the birth is easier and there's less trauma for the little creature.

I won't give you a full run-down on ante-natal exercises, this will be done by your clinic or health visitor, but I'd like to give you the few simple ones that I found most helpful.

BREATHING: Lie on your back on a rug on the floor, with knees bent, and feet flat on the floor.

With the mouth closed, breathe gently in and out, letting the abdominal wall rise up with the indrawn breath and drop down with the outgoing one. This must be practised *every day*, aiming at taking ten seconds to draw in a breath and then gently let it go, gradually reducing the number of breaths per minute.

With the mouth closed, breathe slowly to expand the ribs sideways, opening out the inverted V of the ribs in front. Again let the breath come out gently.

With mouth open, breathe in more quickly, lifting up the sternum or breast bone, and letting it lower again. The mouth is kept open, since during the later part of labour this breathing is used. This type of breathing is shallower and therefore quicker than breathing deeply through the nose. Don't be tempted to do this more often than three times or you will hyper-ventilate (take in too much oxygen) and feel giddy.

RELAXATION: Lie on the floor on one side, head, not shoulders, on a pillow, eyes and mouth gently closed, back and neck well bowed forward, under arm behind the back and bent at the elbow and wrist, top arm also bent lying on the floor (or pillow) in front, top leg should be bent at hip, knee and ankle and placed in front of the bottom leg which is bent in the same manner.

This is usually found to be the most comfortable and effective position for relaxing during pregnancy, because all parts of the body rest on a firm support, so no muscle is tense because it has to work to carry the weight of any part of the body. All joints are loosely bent, so no muscle is unwittingly drawn taut across a joint. (If difficulty is found with the position, put further cushions under any uncomfortable part, but practise on a firm surface.)

Contract and relax each group of muscles in turn, as follows:

Left leg – Squeeze down the toes, relax; bend down the ankle, relax; bend up the ankle, relax; straighten the knee a little way, relax; bend the knee a little way, relax; tighten the hip muscle that you sit on, relax.

Right leg: do the same as with the left leg.

Left arm: stretch the fingers, relax; bend elbow a little way, relax; straighten elbow a little way, relax; tighten the shoulder muscles on which you are lying, relax.

Right arm: do the same as with the left arm.

Face: let all the muscles of face and neck (eyes, mouth, nose, forehead) sag.

When the whole body feels loose and sagging, begin to breathe consciously, naturally and quietly, 'listening' inwardly to what you are doing.

As you breathe, say to yourself, 'in – out', making each word last the appropriate movement of breath. The rhythm of the breathing releases mental tensions and keeping your mind on the 'in – out' prevents any disturbing thoughts from creeping in to destroy the peace of mind which is essential for complete relaxation.

When the relaxation is working the body begins to feel very comfortable, the floor seems soft and you seem to be as light as a feather – finally a feeling of the floor rising up under the body like a lift is experienced. Sleep may, and if the time is right usually will, follow such relaxation. I always fall asleep after this.

The best time to practise relaxation is daily after the midday meal, at the beginning of an afternoon rest and at night when getting ready to go to sleep.

Remember always the three principles of relaxation:

1 Full support for all parts of the body.

2 No muscle tension anywhere – joints, face, hands, feet, etc.

3 Peace of mind.

Once you feel you have acquired some degree of relaxation, try a short period of the breathing described at the beginning of this section since this is the method you will use in the first stage of labour when lying in the relaxation position.

Regaining your figure

It sounds daft, and I suppose I should have realized it, but no one prepared me for the fact that after my baby was born I still looked about seven months pregnant and where that precious little bump had been there were folds of flabby skin. I couldn't believe that it would ever go back into place again, but nature is miraculous and with a little help it does. The help came in the form of a small pamphlet produced by the Obstetric Association of Chartered Physiotherapists. I started some of the exercises the day after birth. You can do them in bed or when you are mobile and home again, on the floor. I still do the tummy pull in and ankle circulation in bed at night.

From the day after birth, do exercises 1 to 4, four times each. From three days onwards do 5 to 7 four times each in addition to original exercises. After a week, increase the exercises to five times each, and after two weeks, do them six times. Keep doing these exercises until you feel able to return to a more strenuous routine.

Every mother differs with regard to regaining her figure – the younger you are, the more supple the skin, still plump with collagen and elastin, and the figure returns quickly. My baby was born mid-May and I was back into a bikini by our holiday in early September. There was a little residual fat here and there but I think I could say I was back to normal within six months. Don't forget, it's essential that you don't put on more than the allowed poundage when pregnant otherwise you'll have the devil's own job losing it. It's a myth that you are eating for two. You should eat normally and wisely for *one*.

Post-natal exercises

1 To freshen stagnant tissues and tone up the tummy, lie with your head on a pillow, knees bent, feet flat. Put your hands half-way down your tummy. Breathe in – feel your tummy go up. Breathe out completely. Pull your tummy wall towards your back, to squeeze out as much air as you can.
2 To tone up legs and circulation, lie with your head on a pillow, legs straight. First bend and stretch ankles. Then point feet upwards. Keep ankles still. Bend and stretch toes. Finally circle feet outwards, and then circle feet inwards.
3 Lying with your head on a pillow, legs straight, press backs of knees and thighs downwards onto bed or floor. Relax.
4 For the pelvic floor muscles, through which a baby is born, lie with your head on a pillow, knees bent and slightly apart, feet flat. Imagine a string attached halfway between your vagina and back passage, running up through your body towards your chin. Now tighten your muscles to pull the string up inside you. Pull up slowly, to the limit. Relax. Feel the pressure *inside*, not round the hips or tummy. Get into

the habit of doing this uplifting movement often – lying on your side in bed, sitting and standing as well.

5 For the waistline, lie with your head on a pillow, one leg bent, the other leg straight. Keep the bent leg still. Make the straight leg shorter by drawing it up from hip and waist. Then make it longer by stretching down. Repeat with the other leg bent.

6 For the front of the tummy, lie with your head on a pillow, knees bent, feet flat. Tighten tummy muscles and pull in. Press waist downwards, hard to round the spine. Keeping waist in contact with bed or floor, lift the hips slightly off it by contracting your buttocks. Relax.

7 For waist and hips, lie with your head on a pillow, knees bent, arms stretched out sideways. Keep feet and shoulders still, knees together. Twisting from waist, swing both knees to touch bed or floor on left, while right hip turns towards ceiling. Then swing knees over to touch on right, while left hip turns towards ceiling.

EXERCISE REMINDER LIST

DON'T get disheartened if you can't do all the exercises in a routine as many times as requested. If it hurts too much or you are breathless, don't push yourself. You will improve with practise. *Don't* overdo it.

DON'T despair if you miss out on a day or two. Rather like dieting, unless you have a life which runs like clockwork, there's always something which might tempt you away from your exercises. Even *once* a week is better than nothing.

DO remember that there are simple exercises you can perform as you go about your everyday life – pulling in tummy muscles while sitting in the car at traffic lights. Loosening your neck, also at traffic lights, particularly if you've had a long journey, your neck can get very stiff.

DO remember exercise tones your heart, increases circulation, aids digestion and excretion, and all in all makes you feel better in mind as well as body.

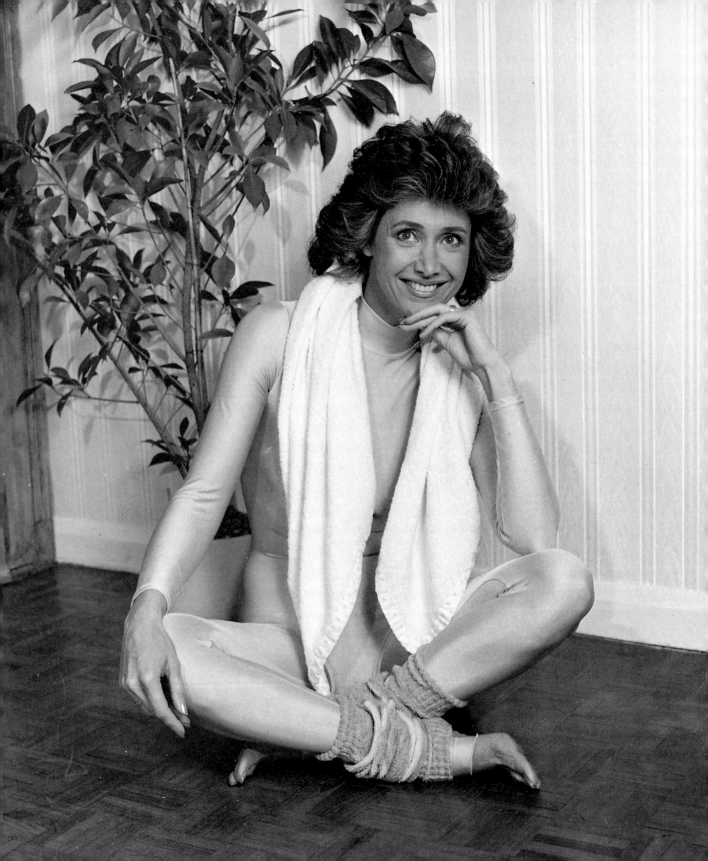

Body Care and Massage

Body care is, of course, a total concept – a balance of the correct nutrition, exercise, relaxation and sleep. You can also give some external help in the shape of massage. Why is it that so few women give a thought to this wonderful therapy? Is it a throwback to the decadent days of Ancient Rome or the association with the 'rich bitch' with nothing better to do than be pampered? If I were in a position to have a retinue of employees at my fingertips, I think I'd choose to have a permanent masseur even before a cleaner and a cook. As it is, I usually only have time for about six massages a year, but that's better than nothing and leaves me with a positive and glowing feeling of relaxation and overall well-being. Obviously it is more beneficial to undergo massage at the hands of an expert, but there's a great deal you can do yourself and should.

Why massage?

Massage comes from the Greek word *massa*, meaning to knead. In fact it's an instinctive reaction – if you get cramp, you automatically massage the painful spot.

Massage tones the skin and improves circulation. This accelerates the removal of waste products in the body via the lymph system. It also inhibits the formation of skintags, warts and cysts. On dry skin, the sebaceous secretion, sebum, is increased, making the skin more supple.

Although massage does not increase *muscle* strength, it does tone muscles. If you are a person who suffers from tension, you will notice how the pain builds up in your muscles, especially shoulder and neck muscles. Massage, properly applied, breaks down these 'tension knots' and alleviates the pain which goes with them. I know, I've sometimes had such pain that I've hardly been able to move my head.

Apart from its therapeutic value, it's heavenly to relax under the hands of a skilful masseur. 'Haven't got the time,' I hear you grumble. Well, a certain amount of time spent looking after yourself pays off. Like a car engine, you can only go on for so long without a service or an overhaul. If you never allow time to overhaul yourself, you will eventually run out of the necessary energy to keep going.

Body massage

It is not easy to give yourself a body massage but there are a few things you can do which are better than nothing at all. You're going to think I've got a fetish about baths because off we go to the bathroom again.

You can give yourself a good invigorating rub every day with one of a multitude of massage gloves on sale – they come made out of loofahs, synthetic fibres, and there is one which you hold like an iron. It has a rubber base with nodules on it and also holes through which the specially formulated soap containing ivy permeates. Any of these used on thighs, hips, buttocks, shoulders – but not stomach or breasts, they are too delicate – will increase circulation and leave the pores of your skin receptive to any creams you choose to put on after your bath. Always apply these with upward strokes – this helps the return of blood to the heart and doesn't drag the skin. Gravity is continually pulling down our skin – don't help it.

You can also knead your flesh with your fingers. Make yourself relaxed to begin with. Get into your warm bath, lie back and stretch your legs out and lift them up as far as they will go comfortably. Lift your arms above your head and stretch. Rather like the movement of a cat – stretch and relax. Now go to your trouble spots, usually thighs and hips. It's probably better if you kneel in the bath, on a rubber mat or face cloth to save your knees. Now, pick up a wad of flesh in your fingertips, hold for a moment, then release – it's almost like a gentle pinching. Keep repeating this action moving about an inch at a time over the trouble spots, waist and upper arms too. It will be more beneficial if you use your right hand for your left side and vice versa – you are then stretching your waist and arm as well. You won't have time for this every day so when you don't, just use your massage glove to create some friction and increase circulation.

Continue your massage out of the bath by using your towel in a massaging movement. Grip ends of the towel in each hand, swing it over your head and dry with a sawing motion over the shoulders, waist, buttocks and thighs.

There are many small massage machines which you can buy in the shops. If you do use one of these, remember to cream your body first with oil or other lubricant and never, never pull the skin. Use gentle circular movements and never be tempted to use a body massaging machine on your face.

Face massage

While taking off your make-up, you've already given yourself a light massage but there are other more specific massage movements for the face and neck.

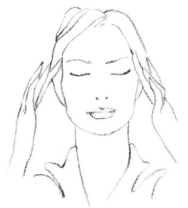

Facial massage
Gently apply pressure to each
temple for a few seconds.

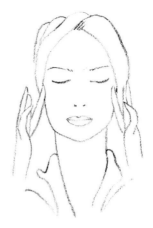

Stroke your middle fingers across
cheek bones.

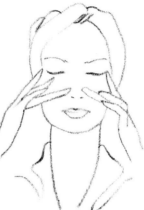

Gently rotate middle fingers at
the corners of the nose.

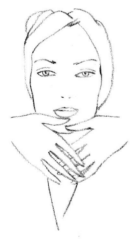

Briskly stroke the chin upwards
with your thumbs, alternating
hands.

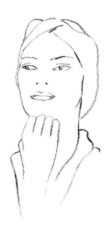

Flick the skin under your chin
with the back of the fingers of
one hand.

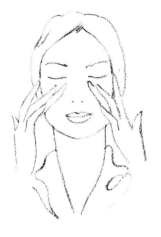

Gently stroke the middle fingers under the eyes, from the outer corner to the bridge of the nose.

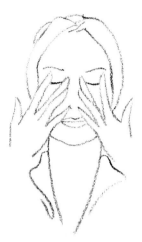

Apply slight pressure at the inner corners of the eyes.

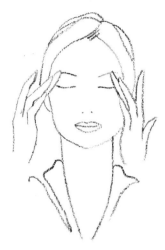

Continue through to stroke the eyebrows round to their outer edge.

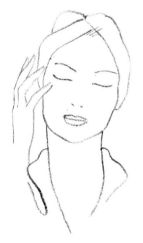

Rotate middle fingers across the forehead from the centre outwards.

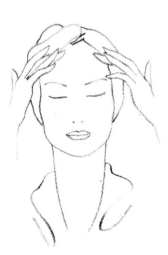

After circling them several times, stroke below the eyes from the outer corner downwards with your little fingers.

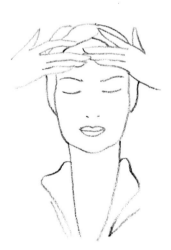

Finally stroke the fingers and palms up across the forehead from the bridge of the nose.

DRY SKIN STROKE MASSAGE: Apply your night-treatment cream. Using the middle finger and forefinger of both hands, barely touch the skin on your face and neck. Move upwards from the neck to the scalp with long, slow strokes. Your fingertips should just brush the fine facial hairs. I hear you asking, how can this possibly be doing any good? It does, by stimulating the nerve endings underneath the skin. It should be done every night. There's nothing to it.

OILY SKIN JACQUET MASSAGE: This massage is named after the French physician who invented it and is intended only for oily skins. Apply your night cream, then with thumb and forefinger lightly pinch the thicker portions of facial skin around cheeks and chin. As you are pinching, lightly rotate the flesh in a half-turn. Some of the oil from your skin is released by this movement. When you have finished, pat your face with cotton wool soaked in water and wrung out. Then dry the face with tissues, again using a patting movement.

THIN SKIN MASSAGE: Fine, thin skin has a tendency to broken capillaries. They're mainly found around the nose and on the cheeks. They are the result of exposure to extremes of temperature, spicy food, alcohol, and, perhaps, rough treatment.

A very gentle tapping massage is good for this condition by creating greater elasticity in the walls of the blood vessels. All you do is gently tap the offending areas with the cushions of your fingers, alternating them as you would when drumming your fingers on a table. I can't do this as well with my left hand as my right so I use the right for both sides of my face. It's amazing to think that such a gentle action is beneficial. You can also take this tapping movement down onto the neck.

NECK MASSAGE: I keep on talking about the importance of neck care, and here is an easy massage which could be combined with your regular night-time beauty routine. Oil the skin lightly, then with flat fingers and palms glide up from collarbone to chin, alternating hands and working up to a steady rhythm. Then reverse hands, as in the diagram which follows, and continue in your rhythm, reversing the hands back and forth until the oil is absorbed.

You can, of course, buy facial massagers. So long as you use them in a gentle fashion, always following the lines of movement recommended here and in the skin care chapter, never pulling the skin, then they are perfectly safe.

Cellulite

Massage helps deal with something the French so delicately call 'cellulite' – which is that unsightly puckered skin, resembling orange peel or cottage cheese, which builds up around too fat thighs, hips, upper arms and insides of knees and ankles.

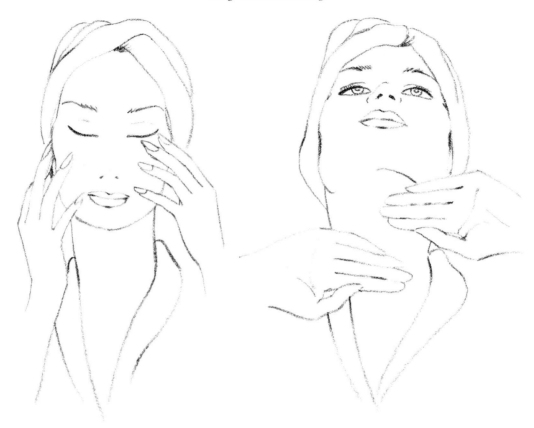

Tapoter
Fast, light tapping on areas blemished by broken veins helps the capillaries to release blockages.

Neck massage
Work up to a steady rhythm on oiled skin, reversing the hands as above from time to time.

Cellulite is narrow filaments of connective tissue packed with globules of fat. This fat sticks to the skin and underlying tissue by a network of fibrous adhesions. With age and weight gain, skin loses its elasticity, it shrinks but the fat cells don't and this causes the dimpling or orange-peel effect. Cellulite does not disappear when you slim and exercise – it requires special treatment. Cellulite is caused by:

POOR CIRCULATION: this may be a genuine medical condition or it can be something self-inflicted by wearing too-tight girdles, to hold in that fat you don't like, and tight trousers.

SEDENTARY OCCUPATIONS: people who spend most of their working life sitting are more likely to suffer from cellulite than those in active occupations.

SHALLOW BREATHING: this may sound odd but there are folk who simply don't take nice deep breaths. Just think, you can live for weeks without food, days without water, but only minutes without air. The air you inhale contains oxygen which breaks down the nutrients you eat to produce energy which nourishes your body cells. Oxygen enters the lungs, fills the tiny bronchioles and then diffuses through them to be carried to every cell in your body. If all this action is not happening efficiently, then toxic wastes build up and, yes, they build up in just the places you don't want them – hips, thighs, etc.

BAD NUTRITION: the wrong foods – too much carbohydrate, starch and fat equals too many calories. And that means fat.

Treatment

1 Salon massage will improve circulation thereby nourishing the cells and shifting the toxic waste – think of the cellulite rather like a blocked drain.
2 Exercise and electrical body treatments.
3 Home massage with a loofah will help but it won't be so effective as professional treatment.
4 Proper nutrition. Alcohol and coffee will have to go if you're really serious about attacking your cellulite. They are major pollutants.
5 Smoking – give it up. It robs your system of vital Vitamin C essential for the collagen in your skin. Nicotine also interferes with circulation so that the feeding and replenishment of your body cells slows down, blocking the drain again and creating ideal conditions for the formation of cellulite.
6 Breathing correctly (see the chapter on Exercise) to clear the system of unwanted substances. Good circulation feeds the cells and gets rid of waste.

Salon massage

If you're going for a professional treatment, let me give you an idea of what to expect. Don't make the mistake that I made in thinking that if I couldn't really 'feel' it, then it was not doing any good. A masseur should never cause you pain. If your muscles are knotted with tension, they will need more time spent on them, but a hard massage that hurts simply isn't on. Always check that the masseur is qualified.

You will find that the therapist uses a combination of movements:

Effleurage   *stroking movements*
Petrissage   *compression movements like kneading bread*
Tapotement   *percussion movements or tapping*

Firm movement is used over muscular or flabby areas such as the tops of thighs, buttocks etc. Light movement is employed over bony areas such as knees and ankles.

Aromatherapy

If I had the time, then I would luxuriate in an aromatherapy massage at least twice a week. What is it? It's a massage using 'essential' oils which are absorbed, primarily through the hair follicles and pores, and in a short space of time find their way into the bloodstream. Essential oils are not like the oils we might immediately think of – olive oil, lanolin, baby oil – they are more like water and are found in tiny droplets in specific parts of plants. They are highly concentrated and before use must be diluted in other oils. Some are so strong they would be capable of burning the skin if used 'neat'. Once absorbed into the skin they are carried by the bloodstream or via the lymph and interstitial fluid (the liquid that surrounds all the body's cells) to other parts of the body.

Essential oils act on different parts of the body. For instance, rose oil has healing properties and appears to have particular influence on the female sexual organs. Lavender and orange blossom oil stimulates the generation of new cells. Fennel oil contains plant hormones similar in structure to oestrogen – mixed with a good carrier oil it can make an anti-wrinkle treatment. Sandalwood oil is good for renal and cardiac deficiencies.

Experiments with animals have shown that when an essence is applied to the skin it reaches an internal organ in half an hour.

The qualities of essential oils were discovered by accident. Years ago, a distinguished French chemist burned his hand badly while working in his laboratory. He spontaneously plunged his hand into a container of pure lavender oil. To his amazement, the hand had virtually healed within a few hours. This led him to do further research and categorization of the healing and cosmetic properties of essential oils. An Austrian biochemist, the late Marguerite Maury, developed a range of aromatherapy beauty treatments where the essential oils were applied to the skin especially along the nerve centres near the spine and on the face. She mixed her oils to suit the individual requirements of each client. Not all salons practising aromatherapy go to these lengths but the oils they use contain substances which are beneficial to all. It's thought that some essential oils extracted from fennel, hops, garlic, ginseng and eucalyptus contain plant hormones which resemble animal hormones and have the ability to revitalise certain organs in the body. The oils also act directly on the skin by encouraging the growth of new healthy cells to replace the dead cells we are shedding constantly.

The oils used in Aromatherapy are extremely expensive which means, unfortunately that the treatments are too.

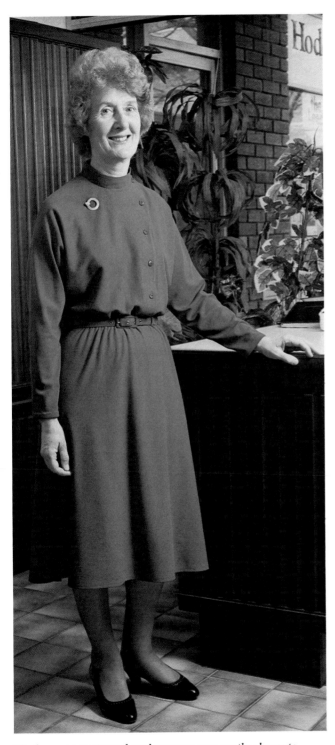

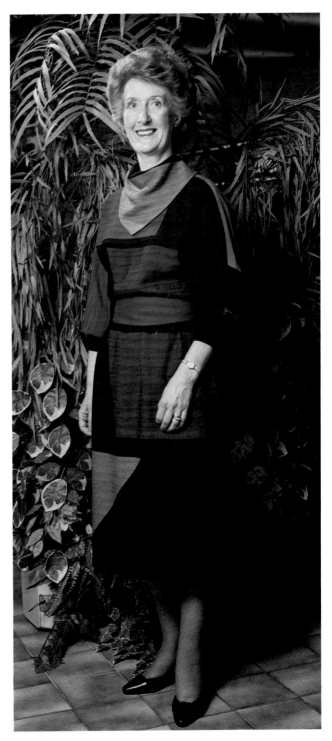

The four women pictured on these pages gave me the chance to give them a completely new look. Having met briefly to choose outfits, we then spent a day at Jean May's Salon near Bristol – my regular hairdresser – where they arrived in clothes and make-up of their choice. Patricia is 38, has two children and is a part-time personal assistant. June is 51 and a part-time secretary. Eva, a housewife, is 57. Pat is a nurse aged 43 and a mother of three.

JUNE We discussed June's new hairstyle and make-up earlier. The attractive blue dress she wore suited her figure but I wanted to see her in warmer colours to complement her red hair and bring out her natural glow. This wool dress has a pretty, scarf-detail neckline which suits her long face. The higher shoes improve the shape of her legs.

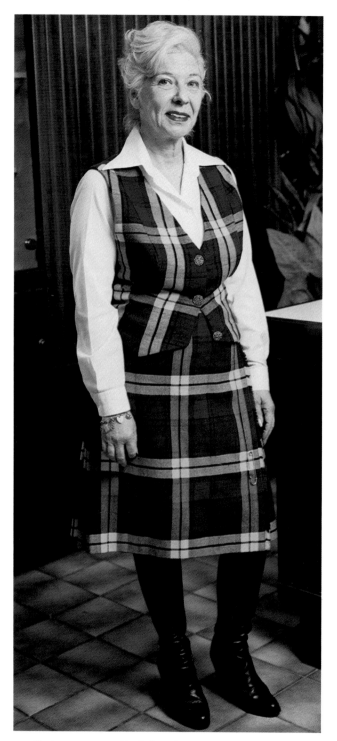

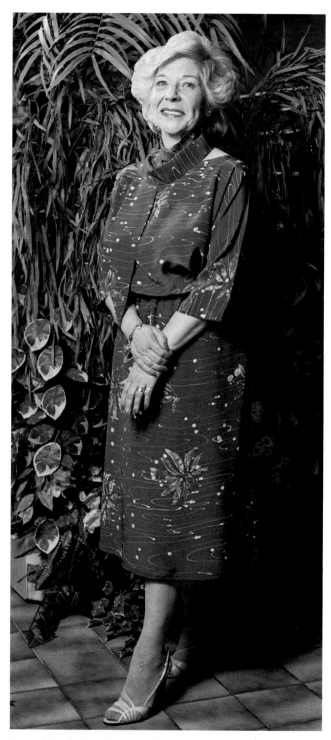

EVA *Tartan accentuates Eva's large bust and the harsh colours make her hair and skin appear sallow. Jean cut her long hair and, using a demi-wave, gave Eva a soft, elegant style. Silver highlights counteracted the yellowing of her grey hair. I gave her olive skin a beige foundation and deep-rose blusher and used grey eye shadow*

to match her hair and outfit, with strong highlight under the brows. Delicate pink lipstick flatters her face far more than her original bright red and picks up the pink in her dress. This is in silk batik – simple and pretty to soften her figure and enhance her colouring. I tied the belt around the neck for extra softness.

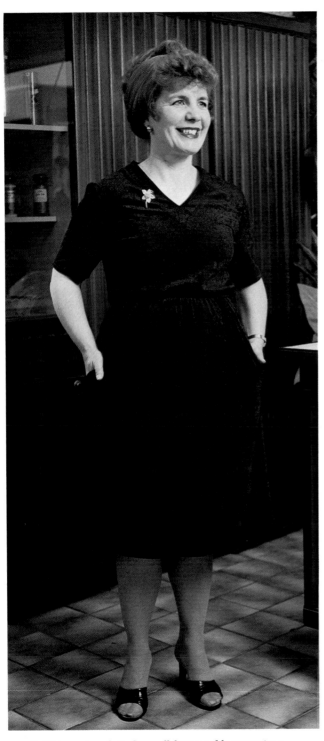

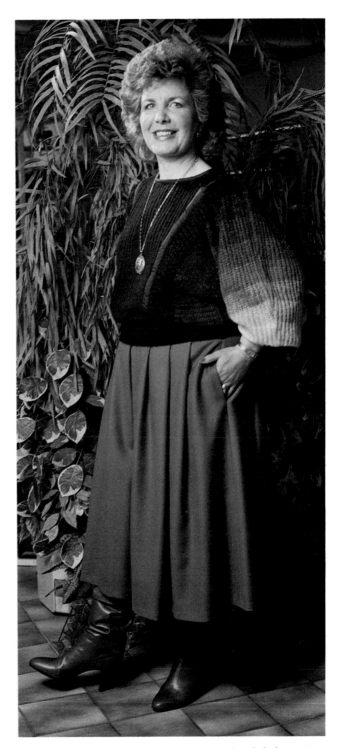

PAT Full hips and a relatively small frame and bust require a balancing act in dressing to avoid looking bottom heavy. Pat's clinging black dress emphasized her figure in the wrong places and had an unflattering neckline. Tied-back hair, a close-fitting bodice and tight sleeves further accentuated her hips and round face. A full hairstyle, with soft shaping make-up (described earlier) help

balance her figure giving width at the head. Gathered clothes are often avoided by full-figured women but these well-cut culottes skim Pat's hips and matched with a loose, batwing sweater give her figure proportion. The boots hold the line of the outfit and make her look taller.

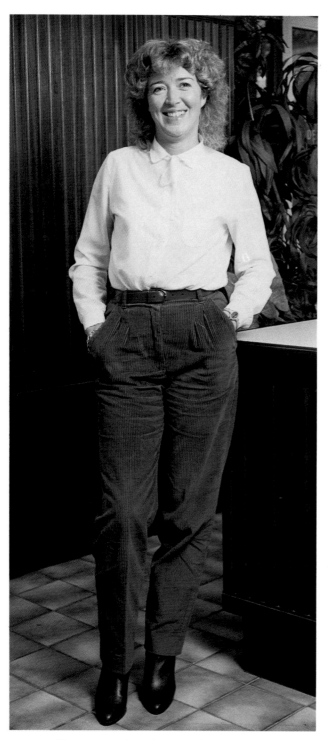

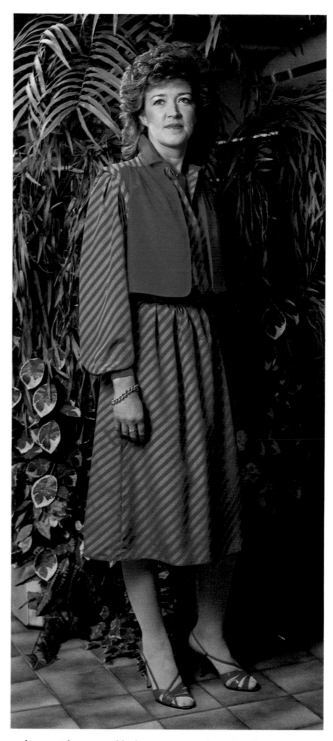

PATRICIA *She was not making the most of her good figure. A close-fitting blouse does not give the width at the shoulders that she needed to go with gathered trousers. Her dull hair was the result of perming and tinting. Jean kept the length at the back but trimmed the sides and swept the hair up and back from the face to give width. The natural-looking colour was achieved with bubble highlights to provide hints of red. I continued this warmth in the* make-up with a tawny blusher over a rosy-beige foundation and a rose lipstick darkened with orangey-red for her new outfit. Her deepset eyes were given grey-blue highlight under the brows, blue pencil and brown cake eyeliner and black mascara. The red and grey dress, with stylish waistcoat and cuff details, suited her beautifully, broadening the shoulders yet soft and feminine with matching strappy sandals.

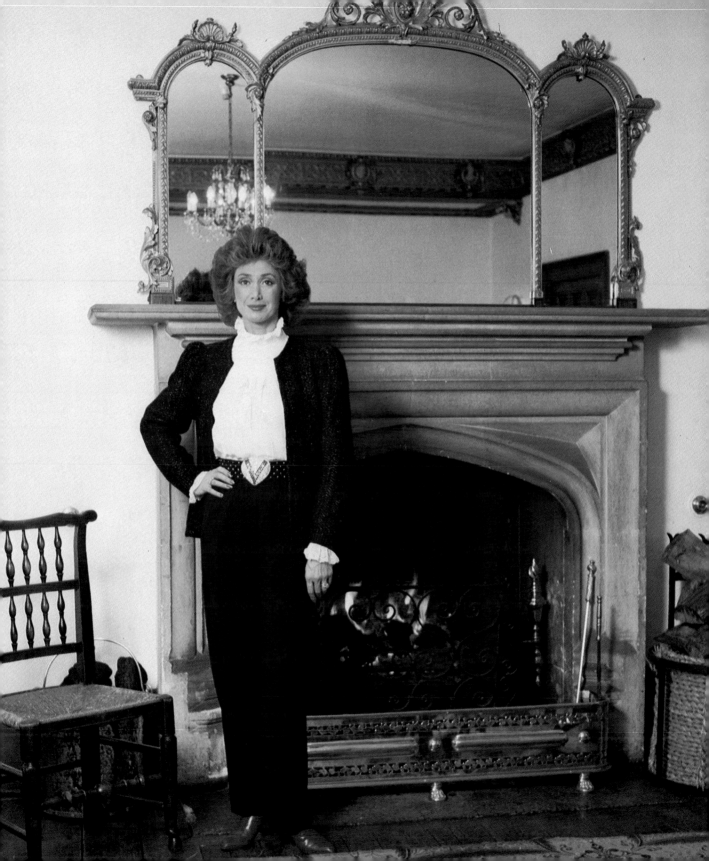

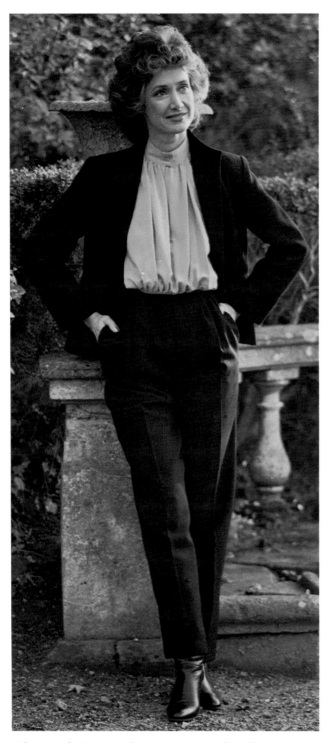

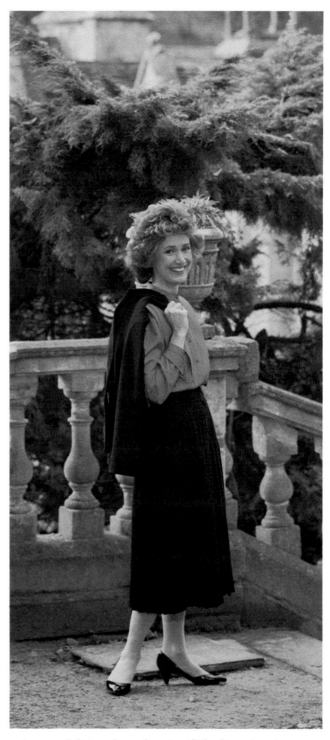

A basic wool suit, or matching separates, is perhaps the most flexible of all clothes. Mine is a co-ordinated outfit – culottes, jacket, trousers and cardigan. I can wear the trouser suit for a daytime appointment and then slip on a lacy blouse, the cardigan

and a pretty belt to make an elegant outfit for dinner (previous page). I find this flexibility essential since I do not always have time to change between appointments and it cuts down on luggage when I am travelling to engagements around the country.

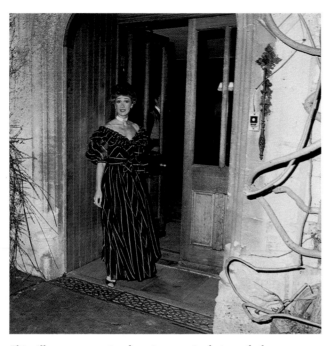

This silk organza evening dress is expensive but worth the investment. Black and white never dates and neither does this classic style – I shall wear it for years.

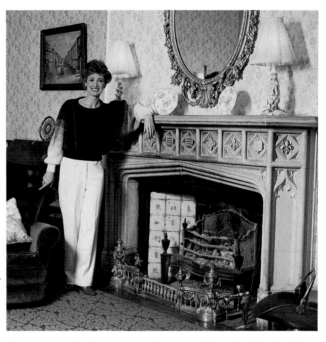

Do you recognize the sweater – it was one I chose for Pat when I gave her a new look and this is a different colour pattern. Batwing sleeves are extremely flattering and soft whilst giving width. The cream wool trousers can be dressed up or left casual as here.

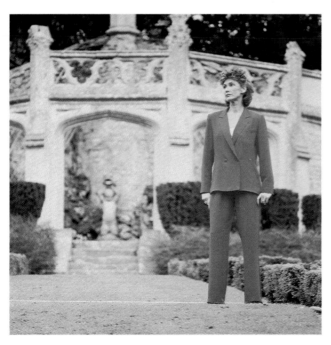

For summer, this well-cut, cherry-red trouser suit, in polyester, is casual enough for the day and the jacket can be slipped off to reveal a pretty camisole for evenings. It is crush-proof, a great bonus, so can be worn for long stretches and easily packed.

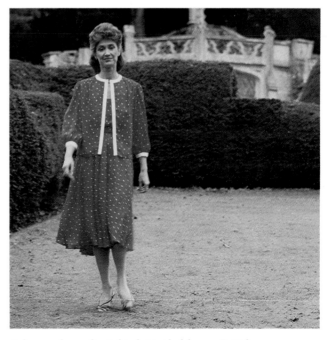

A dress and co-ordinated jacket is ideal for our British summers – giving added warmth when needed without resort to shapeless cardigans or jackets which break the line of the outfit. Again it is crush-proof and pretty, without being too dressy, so meets almost any occasion.

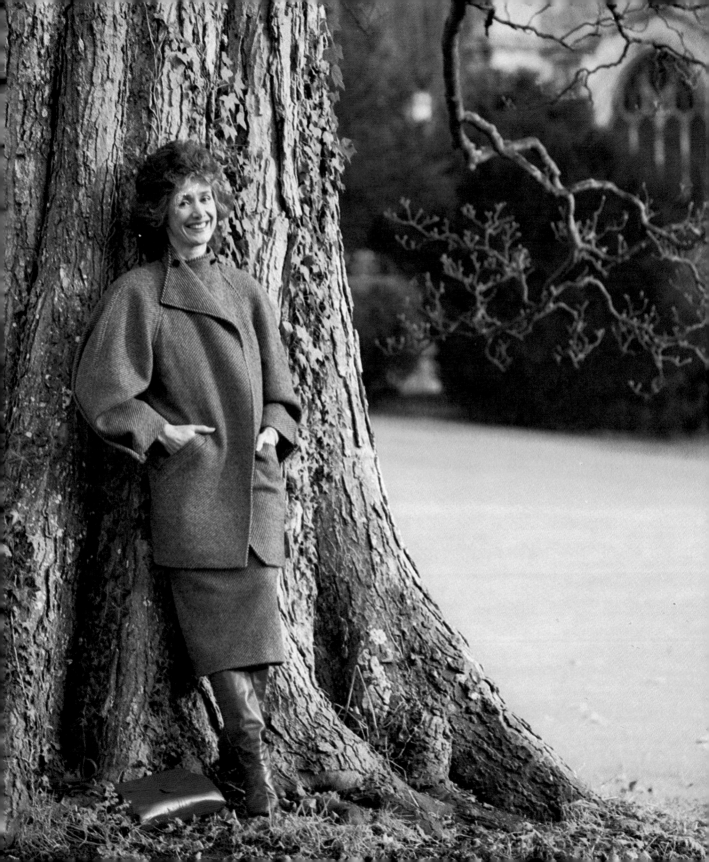

Saunas

These are a very good way of helping clear out the debris from the body by the simple process of sweating. A regular sauna is an aid to controlled dieting and is also helpful in conjunction with a programme of massage to eradicate cellulite. If you suffer from blood pressure, respiratory ailments or heart disease, you should consult your doctor before using a sauna. Never overdo your time in the sauna. If you're new to taking saunas, gently does it.

How does it work?

The sauna has a controlled overheating effect on the body which produces perspiration. You know how salty perspiration is – that's all the impurities coming out of your pores. It increases circulation thus aiding cell renewal. Exfoliation is increased. It has a relaxing and sedative effect on the nerve endings. There is a temporary weight loss but this is quickly restored by the need to drink a lot of fluid after the sauna.

When taking a sauna remember:

1 Leave two hours after your meal before the sauna.

2 Don't stay in the sauna for long periods. Five minutes at a time is perfectly adequate.

3 Take a cold shower after each session and rest before the next.

4 Leave enough time to rest for at least half an hour after your final period in the sauna. That's when you'll probably have a long cool drink and put back the weight you lost in the sauna. Don't worry, you need to replace the water you've lost through sweating.

5 If it is your own home sauna, be sparing with the water on the stones. It's a bit more difficult to regulate this in a public sauna.

If, like me, you feel claustrophobic in a sauna, try a Steam Bath. It has a very similar effect on the body except that your face is outside the cabinet where the temperature of the steam is controlled by the thermostat and adjusted to the needs of the individual.

Body skin care

Caring for the skin on your body is helped enormously by massage and exercise as described – they improve circulation and help rejuvenation. However you can do more. The body skin can be exfoliated in the same way as your face skin, using

This suit is one of my favourites. It is out of the the ordinary, with a three-quarter-length jacket, yet never dates. The full, soft sleeves provide a good contrast to the straight skirt – a flattering and practical combination.

abrasive creams specifically designed for the body. They give you a lovely glowing feeling and keep the skin smooth and toned.

Moisturizing body skin is almost as important as moisturizing your face so use a good, basic body lotion after massaging, bathing or exfoliating. Pay particular attention to dry areas such as knees and elbows.

Rubbing these areas with half a lemon cupped in the hand is also excellent.

Skin care during pregnancy

I started using pre-natal cream from the moment I knew I was pregnant. By the time Jonathan was born I had gone through five pots of the stuff. It is designed to prevent stretch marks and, although some women will get stretch marks come what may, it does help.

Even at my advanced age I was not left with a single stretch mark. You may think that this was due to the fact that I have the sort of skin that doesn't get such marks. In fact I still have stretch marks from my twenties when I was rather plump and then lost weight over a period.

Removing unwanted hair

The legs and underarms of most women are too hairy for their liking but if you are lucky enough to have fine, blonde hair in those places it is best left alone. I had fine, blonde down on my legs until I was convinced, in Australia, that I should remove it. A cameraman there said to me, 'You're a lovely lady, but I wish you'd shave yer legs.' (In broad Australian of course!) Stupidly I did so – and the hair grew back stronger and darker than before. I've been shaving and waxing ever since. The hair on the arms is rarely thick enough to remove. Once removed, the hair will grow back quite quickly and possibly more coarsely.

SHAVING: for legs and underarms, shaving is fine as long as you are prepared to do it regularly and properly. Electric shavers make the whole process a lot easier. Using a wet razor you need a very steady hand, completely clean skin, and to apply a lather of soap first to enable the blade to run smoothly over the skin. Shaving only removes the hair from above the surface of the skin so it will grow again quite quickly.

WAXING: this can be painful the first time you experience it but waxing does remove hair down to the root so it lasts far longer than shaving – up to three weeks before a new hair growth shows. Hot wax applied to the skin can be dangerous and it is definitely best not to attempt it at home but to visit a salon and have it done safely and efficiently by an expert.

Wax strips – more like sticky tape in fact than wax – are now available but my experiments with them have not been too successful. However, if you have fine body hair they can be efficient.

DEPILATION: depilatory creams dissolve the hair just below the surface of the skin. They are perfectly safe, and usually highly effective, provided you follow the instructions on the packet very carefully. Always do a patch test first in case you are allergic to the cream.

Tanning

It is lovely to have a deep tan. For years it has been a sign that one has the wherewithal and the time to lounge around soaking up the sun's rays. However, times are changing and it is not now considered so chic – in fact many women think it's simply stupid to bake your skin to such an extent that you prematurely age it.

I have done more than my fair share of sun worshipping. In my twenties, as I've said, I lived in Australia and was competing with everyone else for the darkest tan on the beach – I wish I hadn't. But then I was unaware of the ravaging effects of the sun. Today, the chic thing to do is *not* get a tan. However, I couldn't go on holiday and stay completely out of the sun – could you? The thing to remember, as I've repeated again and again in this book, is *moderation*.

As you know, the surface of your skin is composed of flattened dead protective cells. Under these are melanocytes, cells which produce a dark pigment when stimulated by the sun's rays. We also have another defence mechanism against the sun and that is the thickening of the dead surface layer – touch your shoulders after days of exposure to the sun, the skin feels hard and leathery and usually this peels first. When the peeling starts we are losing our protective layer, you know how pink the skin is underneath the peel and how sensitive. Although I tan easily and well, I once rather stupidly burnt my shoulders badly. I was on holiday in Corfu and a group of us decided to hire motor scooters and motor over the island – we were all completely fooled by the wonderful breeze we felt as we drove along, forgetting how the sun was mercilessly beating down on our shoulders. I burnt so badly that to this day my shoulders are covered with freckles.

To get a pleasant and safe tan you should follow a few basic rules:

1 Buy a suntan product that will protect your skin and allow the production of pigment to take place slowly. There's no point in rushing at your tan, overdoing it, and then having to stay out of the sun completely for days.

2 You need a stronger sunscreen product for your face than for your body. Your body

is normally clothed and ages less fast than the face. Also too much sun on the face causes wrinkles and broken capilliaries.

3 Don't underestimate the sun, when we get it, even in England.

4 On holiday, begin your tan with only fifteen minutes back and front taken before 11 am and after 3 pm. Why do you think the locals take such long midday siestas – they keep out of the sun when it is at its most fierce and damaging. Increase your sun-bathing, according to your skin type, by five to ten minutes a day, gradually building up your tan.

5 Shower and smother yourself with moisturizing cream at the end of each tanning day. A shower is essential to remove the salt which otherwise irritates the skin.

Hands and feet

Now to probably the most neglected parts of your body – hands and feet. Years ago, most hairdressing salons boasted a manicurist, nowadays they are becoming a rarity – probably because manicuring is labour intensive and therefore uneconomical. So let's do it ourselves.

Nails are formed from hard keratinized cells and their beauty depends on a good diet and protection from damage caused by detergents, household chemicals, too hot water, weather and so on.

Illness and physical conditions can affect the nails – psoriasis, eczema, rheumatism and heart condition will cause ridges and pitting. Stress over a prolonged period manifests itself in vertical lines down the nails, particularly on the little fingers. Splitting and breaking occurs because of a lack of Vitamin A. Women who are on the pill very often suffer white spots and white lining on the nails due to a deficiency of Vitamin B6. Damage is also done to the nails by incorrect filing and by digging into the cuticles during a manicure. I know a lot of women complain that they don't like wearing gloves for housework but you really should wear them for washing up. You must use gloves when gardening, and you should also protect your hands from the cold in winter. Feet are probably the Cinderella factor in the body, but hands run them a close second. We forget that we should moisturize, protect and cosset our hands. And those unsightly brown age spots can be kept at bay if you put some ultraviolet screening cream on your hands when the sun is shining.

Massage is important for the hands and nails.

Manicure equipment

VARNISH REMOVER: Oil-based

CUTICLE CREAM: To soften and nourish the cuticle

CUTICLE REMOVER: To loosen and release the cuticle which adheres to the nail.

PASTE POLISH: This is used with a nail buffer on ridged uneven, or lifeless nails, or where no nail varnish is used. Blood supply to the nail is increased by the buffing action.

NAIL WHITE PENCIL: An optional extra used to whiten the free edge of the nail. The pencil is wetted before use.

BASE AND TOP COATS: These play an important role in prolonging the life of the varnish. More important, the base coat helps prevent staining from the varnish and smoothes over the small ridges and pits in the nail. Some women who use nail varnish constantly, end up with a handful of what look like nicotine-stained finger-nails. Very ugly.

NAIL STRENGTHENERS: If your nails are less than perfect, a strengthener will help treat brittleness and fragility.

HAND CREAM: To moisturize

EMERY BOARDS: Extra long ones

ORANGE STICKS

SMALL BOWL OF WARM WATER

Hand manicure

1 Remove old varnish with cotton wool soaked with remover. Always wipe away from the cuticle otherwise varnish and remover can be swept under the cuticle where it can be damaging. If there is any stubborn polish around the nail edges and cuticle, use an orange stick wrapped in cotton wool and soaked in remover.
2 Using a long emery-board on the fine side, file the nails from edge to centre. Never saw at your nails – this causes friction on the nail surface and leads to splitting. Don't file too low down at the sides of the nail.
3 Massage cuticle cream into the nails and cuticles. Place hands in water for a few minutes.

4 Dry hands and then, with a cotton-wool-tipped orange stick, put cuticle remover around cuticles. Gently push back the cuticles. It is a good idea to get into the habit of pushing back the cuticles whenever the hands have been in water. Don't trim the cuticles unless it is absolutely necessary – they will grow back even thicker.

5 Apply hand cream, massaging from the fingers to the wrist and up the arm about five inches. Using the thumb, massage the palm with a circular movement.

6 Remove the hand cream from the nails with a light wipe of cotton wool soaked in remover.

7 Apply the nail strengthener if used and then the base coat (as shown in diagram) using light fast strokes for even coverage.

8 Apply varnish as shown, using two coats. If a darker shade is required you can add a third coat but remember it takes much longer to dry.

9 Apply top coat to finish.

10 Apply drying solution if required. This is available in spray or liquid form.

Pedicure

This is simply a manicure for the feet. The only extra implement you will need is a pair of good toenail clippers. Follow the instructions as for a manicure except for 2 – here instead of using an emery-board, you should cut your toenails straight across with the clippers, no shorter than the end of the toe. Never shape your toenails. Use hand cream to moisturize as you would for your hands. For any corns or stubborn hard skin, go to a chiropodist for treatment, don't dig around with razors and the like. Chiropodists are not desperately expensive and even the worst feet only need treating about twice a year. It's quite refreshing to add a tablespoon of washing-soda and a handful of herbs – mint, lavender, rosemary – to the warm water in which you soak your feet.

Nail varnish application

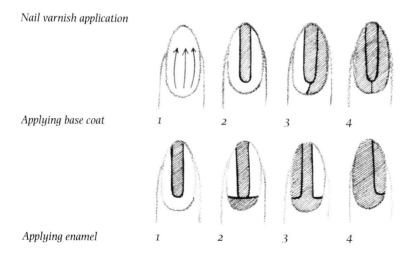

Applying base coat   *1*   *2*   *3*   *4*

Applying enamel   *1*   *2*   *3*   *4*

While your varnish is drying why not lie on your bed or the floor with your feet higher than your head. I usually lie back with my posterior as close to the head-board as I can get it and then stick my legs up the wall. This relieves the feet and legs and is most relaxing. I do this if I've had a hard day and have a quick turn around to go out for the evening. A nap is out of the question, but if your legs and feet are rested it certainly gives you a top-up of energy.

Feet are a neglected part of the anatomy and yet rested feet can give one a feeling of well-being. One's feet should also be supple. Here are a few simple exercises: –

1 Roll an unopened tin under the feet from the toes to the heels.
2 Pick up a pencil with the toes. Easier said than done!
3 Flex the toes by stretching and then relaxing them.
4 Curl the toes under tightly and then relax.
5 Rotate the feet first one way then the other. Do these exercises about five times each. Also, try and go barefoot as much as possible.

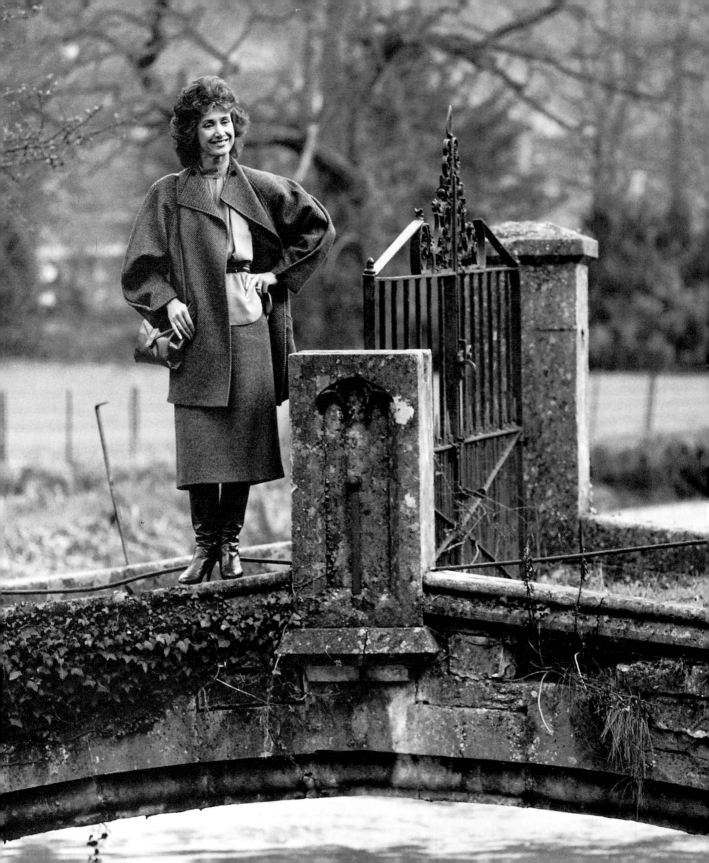

Clothes and Style

Clothes are an extension of one's personality. It is therefore difficult to give advice unless one knows a person intimately and understands what they are all about. However, I do think it's possible to give helpful tips which any woman can consider when she's buying her wardrobe. My number one maxim has always been *quality* rather than quantity. I also believe that clothes are meant to *enhance* the body not draw attention to its faults.

I like an integrated wardrobe – by that I mean when you've found a shop range or designer whose clothes suit your requirements, figure and cheque-book, stay with them. I get bored and flustered going from shop to shop, stripping off, trying on, and dressing again. In the end I've often bought something out of desperation, a garment light years away from what I'd gone out to get and something of which I tired quickly. I find it easier to frequent the same shops – you know the makes they stock and what to expect and often the sales staff get to know you and will, if you're a regular, put garments on one side when new stock arrives and give you a phone call to let you know the new season's wear is in.

It sounds daft but if you want the pick of the new season you need to shop unseasonably. Don't wait until winter has got us in its icy-fingered grip before shooting off for some winter clothes. The best will have gone. Rather like the poor models who have to model coats in summer and bikinis in winter, for winter you need to go shopping when it's still relatively warm, sometimes downright hot, in August and early September.

The same applies to summer wear. Try buying some nice clothes to take on holiday in July – the best went in March and April. Of course shops get deliveries other than just three months in the year but if you did see something you liked but not in your size, early in the season, it could probably still be ordered. Later on you've no chance.

The whole fashion world may seem to work in total disarray and entirely independently. In fact the colours for the season are decided upon by the leading designers and the chain stores follow suit. The accessory manufacturers also 'go with' the season's colours – as you will know to your cost if you've ever tried to buy a particular colour of shoe and handbag which is not in vogue at the time. I like grey accessories and have to buy them and store them when they're available for they too go in and out of fashion. I suppose the only four colours you will always be able to purchase are the basic black and brown, beige and white shoes and handbags.

One summer, there were a lot of what I call 'ice-cream' colours – delicate yellows, pinks, and the palest turquoise. I thought I would never find matching accessories but of course I did because the accessory market works hand in glove with the fashion world. However, I doubt that I'll be able to buy pale turquoise shoes this year!

I don't believe in following fashion slavishly. Few women can carry off the extremes of fashion or have the wherewithal to afford it. One can adapt the best of the current fashion to suit oneself. I happen to like dresses and blouses with a high neckline, preferably frilled. That line was in fashion a while ago, so I bought an extra couple of blouses to hoard against the time when I can't buy them. I have quite a few clothes that are trotted out in my private life year in and year out – I don't wear them on television because somehow the public expects me to change my clothes seasonally. Evening dresses are too expensive to be discarded after a season. I keep them and my oldest and most favourite is just celebrating its ninth birthday. It was a classic when I bought it and still is.

Some women are fortunate enough to be able to buy a whole new wardrobe every season but they are very much in the minority. Most of us 'top up' our wardrobes and the most sensible way to do that is to make a list of what you've already got and take it with you when you shop. Then, if you see a beautiful blouse which is more than you wanted to outlay, but you know you can team it up with a pair of last year's trousers or a skirt, you can indulge because that's all you have to spend. Shopping gets expensive when you buy something on impulse and then realize you haven't a darned thing to go with it – no shoes, no handbag, and your coat won't go over the bat-wing sleeves! Try not to impulse buy because the only time this works is when you see something and you know, *simply know* that it will fit into your wardrobe – the suit you don't need *now* but know you won't be able to find when you *do* want it.

It's a great temptation, but try not to shop if you're feeling low – you'll make mistakes and probably end up loathing the thing. Be wary of sales. The very fact that you're getting a bargain can tip the balance between a buy that is good for you and one that isn't really necessary.

Choosing your wardrobe

Winter

As one who almost lived in unmitigated blacks and browns for years as a leftover from the days when I was fat, do go for some colour. I have only discovered the joy of colour in the last few years.

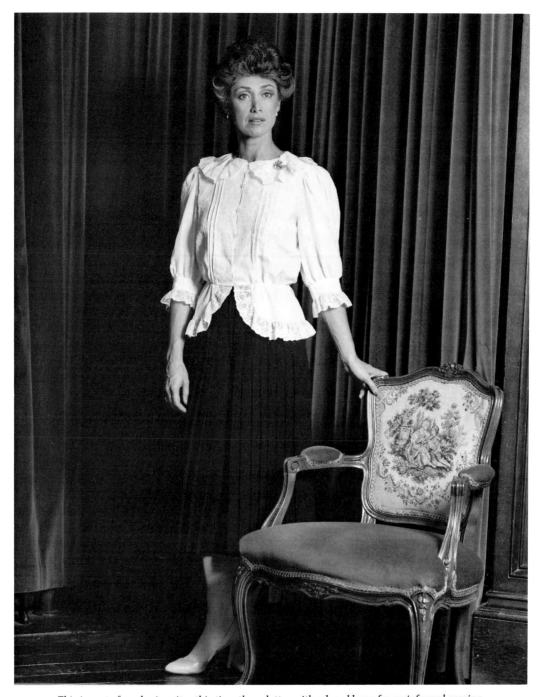

This is part of my basic suit – this time the culottes with a lacy blouse for an informal evening.

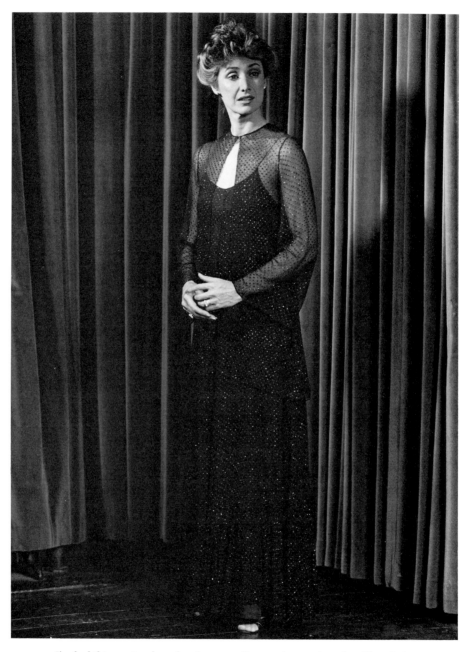

I've had this evening dress for nine years. It seemed expensive when I bought it but the use – and compliments – I've had for it proves its worth.

People were always saying that I'd look good in red, a colour I used to dislike intensely, and they were correct. It does look good and it's well-nigh impossible to feel down when you're wearing such a gay colour. Many women veer away from colours because they are worried about the cost of matching accessories. Don't be. In the winter, grey goes with just about everything except brown. Of course, the little black shoes and handbag are good to have in the wardrobe but I think black is the obvious *easy* option.

CO-ORDINATES: a less expensive way of filling the wardrobe because you can mix and match (provided you take that clothes list with you wherever you go to shop).

A CLASSIC SUIT: a must if you lead a busy life and have to go on from work to an evening engagement. The suit can be transformed with the addition of a feminine and frilly lace blouse or a glitter top or even some chunky jewellery.

A VELVET JACKET: I always have one in my wardrobe – that too can transform an ordinary working skirt and blouse into something smarter and it looks good worn over a dress. Again don't go for the obvious black or brown – burgundy or dark green goes with almost everything and they are colours that suit most women.

A DRESS OR TWO: If you're a working girl and travelling and sitting a lot, go for the fuller skirted dress – it creases less.

WHAT ABOUT FABRIC? Well, I must admit to not liking man-made fibres though sometimes it's difficult, not to mention expensive, to get away from them. If you can't afford wools, go for the best in the man-made line – cheap ones don't wear well, wash or clean well, and don't look good for long. Mixes of natural fibres and man-made will probably give you the best wear. Silk, although luxurious and sought after is the devil to maintain – it creases badly and has to be dry-cleaned. I find silk and polyester mixes wear better.

WINTER COAT: these days there's no absolute necessity for a winter coat because so many people drive and a full-length coat is not at all comfortable in a car. However, when you're choosing your coat, remember that it has to go over layers of clothing so, unless you're incredibly slim, I would suggest that you steer away from the belted variety. A Raglan sleeve is also a much better buy because it will easily go over your outer clothes including a jacket or suit.

UNDERWEAR: whether you are small, medium, or large around the bosom you need a good bra. That doesn't mean expensive, it just means a bra that fits well. Most large stores have in the lingerie department an assistant trained to help you buy the right bra. For a basic wardrobe I'd suggest going for dark shades (white looks so tatty in winter no matter how careful you are with the washing) and also at least one flesh-coloured set for your more diaphanous blouses. Nothing looks worse than a pretty blouse with a bra shining through it like a flashing Belisha beacon.

Summer

A JACKET: an absolute must is a white, beige, or neutral jacket. A cardy over a summer dress totally ruins your image, unless it's cashmere and that's a bit warm. In this climate of ours we don't often get the opportunity to prance around in skimpy summer dresses. Invariably some extra protection is needed and how many summer nights can you think of where you didn't need a wrap of some sort. I have a white tailored jacket which I bought in a large department store and it's now entering it's third summer. Yes, it does have to be cleaned frequently but at least it looks smart over summer clothes.

SKIRTS: cotton or linen but not straight because of creasing. These can be teamed with more formal blouses if you're a working girl and tee-shirts for casual wear. Your jacket will complement this outfit.

DRESSES: it's good to have at least one dress in the wardrobe, preferably full-skirted. On the rare warm days we do get, straight skirts are hot to wear and don't look good without tights and a decent pair of shoes. A floaty full skirt can easily be worn with bare legs and sandals. Do be careful about the sleeves though. Very few women have good enough arms and shoulders to take sleeveless dresses. They can be fore-shortening and unflattering. A sleeve down to the elbow is becoming to most women.

TROUSERS: when choosing your trousers remember that pure cotton creases badly. A cotton and polyester mix will give you better wear. Linen trousers are lovely for summer wear but they need to be cleaned because only the dry-cleaner can put the dressing back into them.

ACCESSORIES: white shoes and handbag are the easy option but they do go with everything. A pair of flattish casual shoes is always useful. If you have a well-co-ordinated wardrobe buy pastel accessories.

SWIMWEAR: take a good look at yourself in the mirror wearing only bra and pants. Be brutally truthful with yourself – have you got the figure for a bikini or not. If not, then go for one of those incredibly sexy one-piece swimsuits. In fact, to be perfectly honest, I think the one-piece suit flatters every woman better than a bikini but most of us want to get as much as possible of our body tanned – with caution don't forget.

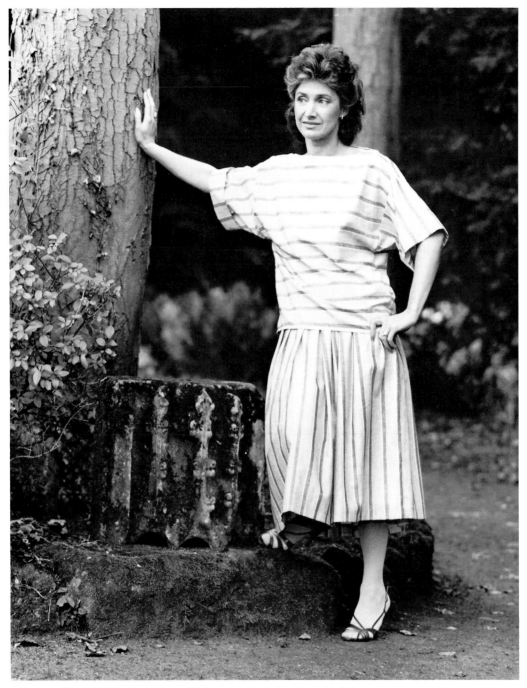

A loose and cool two-piece, which can of course be split up, for informal summer occasions.

127

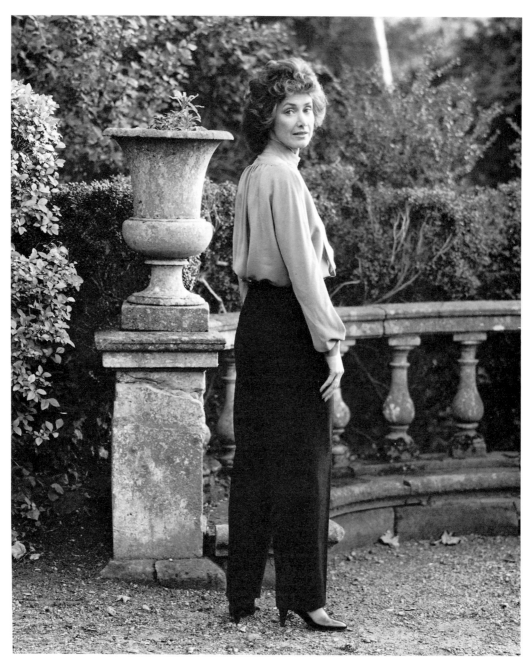

I never wear tight jeans – they do nothing for my figure. These black wool trousers are beautifully cut to skim the hips and taper to the ankle and have a flattering high waist. They're also part of my basic suit.

Do buy a matching wraparound. I know they're not cheap but you've got an instant outfit for lunching on holiday or wandering down to the local shops. The other good thing about the matching wraparound is that you can cover up parts of your body which have had their fair share of the sun if you still want to sit on the beach.

SUN-DRESS: people don't seem to dress in the evenings any more when they are on holiday. A cotton sun-dress will take you to dinner and the disco.

CLOTHES DO'S AND DON'TS

DO buy quality rather than quantity. You'll get far more benefit from a quality garment – it looks better, feels better, wears better and cleans better.

DO remember to take that list of your other clothes with you when you shop.

DO buy good quality matching accessories. It's better to have one good set than a jumble of cheap ones. A good leather handbag will last for years – shoes, well, that depends on how you wear them and of course shoes do date quicker than handbags.

DO (and I'll probably be shot for suggesting this) grab a handful of the material of a potential purchase to see how crease resistant it is. Nothing is worse than buying an outfit, wearing it and looking as though you've slept in it. Sometimes the most expensive fabrics crease badly – silk, cotton and linen – unless they have a man-made fibre mixed with them.

DO take a good look when buying a bikini or swimsuit. Make sure it isn't cut too high at the back so that it rides over that little roll most of us have between buttocks and thighs. Here again, a more expensive item of swimwear won't be skimped and will tuck into your behind in a flattering manner.

DO think tall. Hold yourself erect, don't slouch. You'll look better in the clothes you wear and feel better because you're not squashing your lungs and putting a strain on your back.

DO remember that well-chosen clothes 'do' something for you, and for your figure.

DON'T go for heavy floral patterns if you are short or fatter than you would like to be.

DON'T go for vertical lines if you are tall.

DON'T buy clothes which are not easy to wear. Your clothes should flow on you, not restrict you.

DON'T wear skirts above the knee if you're past your middle twenties, whatever the fashion. On the knee or below it is the most flattering length for you.

DON'T wear flat shoes if you have thick legs and ankles. A slight heel will give your leg a better line.

DON'T wear solid white shoes if you have big feet. Strappy sandals are all right. And don't wear dark tights with white shoes – you'll look like Minnie Mouse!

DON'T forget to create an illusion if you're not as slim as you would like to be. Wear looser clothing. Don't wear clingy acrylics.

DON'T forget to lift dark clothing with coloured accessories – belt, scarf, jewellery.

The Last Word

I hope that the previous chapters will help to make you healthier and more attractive. But the real 'beauty' will have to come from within you. You've heard people remark that someone has 'an inner glow' and that is what it's all about. How often have you been at a gathering and seen people clustered around a woman, not the prettiest in the room, nor the most glamorous, nor the youngest, not the best dressed, but she has a magnetism that defies description. It comes from knowing exactly who you are, what you are, and what your limitations are; from minimizing the bad points and maximizing the good points in one's character. It comes from a *positive attitude* to life.

There is no point in wasting precious time bemoaning what you aren't or what you haven't got. Be aware of what you *are* and what you have got. Not everyone can get to the top of the ladder and not everyone wants to. If you are a woman running a successful home and marriage who feels slightly out of things socially because your areas of conversation are limited in company, then go and get an interest, find a subject that absorbs you and read about it. Go to night school, become an expert on what you find interesting and others will be interested too. When the working woman declares she envies you the time you have to indulge in art classes or cooking cakes she's not looking down at you – she means it. None of us can have our cake and eat it, we all miss out on some things.

Discover who you are, how you feel, and what you want out of life. This isn't selfishness. If you bend your needs and desires to fit in with everyone else, you're not a proper person. That doesn't mean riding roughshod over people either. You must be accountable for your own life and your own actions. Nothing and no one on God's earth can *make* anyone do anything. How often do we moan that it was 'so-and-so's' fault – that man broke my heart, that woman got the job I should have got. That man didn't break your heart – you allowed him to break it. That woman got the job because she was better than you – tough, better luck next time.

Respect yourself, like yourself, and do what *you* want. Be responsible for yourself. Accepting personal accountability for your life actually puts you in control of it.

Believe me, I should know, because I've committed every mistake in the book. 'Life isn't fair,' I'd say. No, it jolly well isn't, and the sooner you realize it the better. You get out of life what you put into it. That's why the outgoing woman who gives of herself gets so much back. I have a very dear friend some twenty years older than myself. She is a large but beautiful woman and everybody loves her – I have never heard a bad word uttered about her. Her life has been no bed of roses but she is a giver and her otherwise empty life is absolutely filled with friends – not acquaint-ances, but friends. I have never heard her bemoan her lot or blame others – her attitude to life is utterly positive.

My attitude to life changed somewhat after a deep conversation at a party with a psychoanalyst. Poor man, what a busman's holiday. Let me tell you, briefly, his advice. He suggested that if you didn't love yourself, how could you expect others to love you. He was the one who pointed out that we are all totally responsible for our actions and though we might think someone else is pulling the strings, they will only do so if we let them. He also said that you should: never say sorry; never make excuses for yourself; and never regret your actions. By that he didn't mean that we should all be rough and abusive but rather that before we act, we should consider the consequences so that we don't have to regret, make excuses or apologize.

We must all learn the wisdom of gracious acceptance – accepting the life that lies between our aspirations and limitations. Never look back either, for yesterday is gone forever and tomorrow marks the beginning of the rest of your life.

Further Reading

Arpel, Adrien *How to Look Ten Years Younger* (Judy Piatkus, London, 1980)
Hudson, Clare Maxwell *The Natural Beauty Book* (Macdonald, London, 1976)
Hunter, Celia *Positive Beauty* (Hutchinson, London, 1980)
Kenton, Leslie *The Joy of Beauty* (Century, London, 1983)
Slimming Magazine *Slimming: The Complete Guide* (Collins, London, 1982)
Voak, Sally Ann *The She Book of Beauty* (Arthur Barker, London, 1979)

Picture Acknowledgments

The photographs on the pages listed below are reproduced in this book by kind permission of the following:

BBC copyright: 10 *below left* and 59 *right*
Harlech Television: 59 *left* and 88 *right*
Jan Leeming: 6, 10 *above left* (photograph by Roy Melhuish), 57 *left* (photograph by Vigo Taurins), 57 *right*, 58 *right* and 88 *left* (both photographs by R. Carpenter Turner)
Sunday Mirror: 4
Weidenfeld (Publishers) Ltd/Edward St Maur: ii, viii, 12, 40, 43, 54, 70, 90, 104, 120, 123, 127, 128 and all the colour photography

The author and publisher also thank Mrs Ed Kyle-Price for allowing the photographs on colour pages 1–4 to be taken in her home; the Manor House Hotel, Castle Combe, Wiltshire for allowing the photographs on colour pages 13–16, and on pages 120, 123, 127 and 128, to be taken in the hotel and grounds; and to Jean Mays for allowing the photographs on colour pages 5, 6 and 9–12 to be taken at her salon in Portishead, Avon.

Clothes for June, Pat, Eva and Patricia were supplied by Leokadia of Bristol, and shoes by Fenice. June's dress is by Infinitif of Paris; Pat's culottes are by Infinitif of Paris and sweater by Oui of Germany; Eva's dress is by Bentley and Spens; Patricia's dress is by Serge Nancel of Paris. Jan Leeming's clothes in the colour photographs are all by Parigi, except for the long dress by Gina Fratini, the tweed suit by Monica Chong and the bat-wing sweater by Oui of Germany.

Index